The Foundations of
INTEGRATED CARE

Facing

the

Challenges of

Change

MARJORIE A. SATINSKY

 American Hospital Publishing, Inc.
An American Hospital Association company
Chicago

This publication is designed to provide accurate and authoritative information in regard to the subject matter covered. It is sold with the understanding that neither the author nor the publisher is engaged in rendering legal, accounting, or other professional service. If legal advice or other expert assistance is required, the services of a competent professional should be sought.

The views expressed in this publication are strictly those of the authors and do not necessarily represent official positions of the American Hospital Association.

ⓐ is a service mark of the American Hospital Association used under license by American Hospital Publishing, Inc.

Cover design by Tim Kaage

Library of Congress Cataloging-in-Publication Data

Satinsky, Marjorie A.
    The foundations of integrated care: facing the challenges of
change / Marjorie A. Satinsky.
        p.   cm.
    Includes bibliographical references and index.
    ISBN 1-55648-207-8 (hard cover)
    1. Integrated delivery of health care—United States. 2. Health
services administration—United States. I. Title
    [DNLM: 1. Delivery of Health Care, Integrated—organization &
administration—United States.   W 84 AA1 S18f 1997]
    RA971.S28 1997
    362.1'068—dc21
    DNLM/DLC
    for Library of Congress   97-17763
                                                CIP

ISBN: 1-55648-207-8   Item Number: 015300

CONTENTS

ABOUT THE AUTHOR

Marjorie A. Satinsky, MBA, FACHE, is executive director for ReXMeD, a physician-hospital organization in Raleigh, NC. She has held senior managed care positions at Duke University Medical Center & Health System in Durham, NC; The Malden Hospital in Malden, MA; and the North Shore Medical Center in Salem, MA. She is an adjunct lecturer for the Department of Health Policy and Administration, School of Public Health, University of North Carolina at Chapel Hill, and a guest lecturer at the Duke University School of Nursing, in Durham.

INTRODUCTION

I f statistics are valid, integrated health care delivery and financing systems are spreading across the United States like kudzu in an untended southern garden. According to a national health care consultant, in April 1995, there were 430 "integrated health networks"—an increase of 69 percent over the number of networks in December 1994 (Shriver 1995). In spring 1996, a nationally recognized expert predicted that the number of systems would grow to 1,200 by the year 2000 (Sokolov 1996).

None of the stakeholders in health care—that is, patients, providers, insurers, and suppliers—have been immune to integration. In the hospital industry alone, 43 mergers and acquisitions occurred in the third quarter of 1995 (Much ado 1996). Nine of those deals involved one large national for-profit company, Columbia/HCA. The growth of Premier, the country's largest alliance, brought that organization to include almost one-third of all hospital beds in the country (News at deadline 1996; Yandell 1997).

Physicians, too, have experienced changes in the organization of their practices. To retain existing business and gain more, many physicians have merged practices and/or sought the security of purchase and management by physician management companies, hospitals, and health care systems.

Integration in the health care industry has not been restricted to providers. Health plans and insurers have joined forces with each other and with providers. Integration on the supply side, particularly in the pharmaceutical industry, has been frenetic (Kropko 1996).

On a national scale, the list of integration participants has been impressive. Although the highly publicized potential alliance between WellPoint Health Networks and Health Systems International did not materialize in 1995, both large health plans pursued relationships with other partners. WellPoint later announced plans to buy the health subsidiary of Massachusetts Mutual Life Insurance Company and the health insurance products of John Hancock Mutual Life Insurance Company. Long-time West Coast competitors PacifiCare Health Systems and FHP International, Inc., combined resources (PacifiCare 1996). Then Foundation Health Corporation and Health Systems International entered into merger discussions and created a new company, Foundation Health Systems, Inc.

There has been similar activity in the insurance industry. Travelers and Metropolitan Life, two of the country's largest insurance companies, joined forces with each other; United HealthCare Corporation then purchased MetraHealth Companies for $1.7 billion. In spring 1996, Aetna Life and Casualty Company acquired U.S. Healthcare HMO for $8.9 million (Kertesz 1996). In an arrangement watched closely by the entire health care industry, Blue Cross and Blue Shield of Ohio and for-profit giant Columbia/HCA attempted to forge a partnership (Findlay 1996; Lutz 1996).

These statistics and activities are misleading because they imply that integration within the health care delivery system, with and without insurance and/or supplier components, is a sure thing that will add value for consumers, payers, and providers. There are, however, reasons to doubt that the trends in integration will continue, that all integration start-up efforts will culminate in viable systems, and that the many integration efforts sweeping the country will be worth the time, effort, and dollars devoted to them.

Creating, operating, and sustaining integrated systems are complex and costly activities that parallel establishing and running a large conglomerate in the non-health-care world. Integrated systems that are provider-controlled have performed less well financially than the rest of the managed care industry. Although the number of systems has continued to grow, many systems have failed (Lessons 1996). Given the public acclaim over systems, dramatically little proof of their value has been demonstrated. It is possible that the market may not want what the supply side is creating (Advisory Board 1995, 151).

My perspective on integrated health care systems is from the inside looking out. As director of managed care contracting/operations at Duke University Medical Center & Health System, Durham, N.C., I have had the opportunity to participate in the start-up of an integrated health system created by a strong academic medical center.

Although my perceptions about integrated systems are from the inside, my conclusions are not dissimilar from those of the researchers and consultants who have examined and worked with systems from the outside. I see many positive qualities in organizations that call themselves integrated health care systems. Many take seriously the health of the communities that they serve. Some really do plan ahead, articulating a mission and objectives that are clearly communicated throughout the system. Some systems realize that values and corporate culture, along with structure, must change. Astute systems, not the majority, concentrate on clinical integration. A handful have the leadership needed to make it happen.

So I am skeptical. I share Stephen Shortell's observation that most integrated systems develop because their component parts, not the market, "will them into being." I see mergers and acquisitions that never progress beyond the signatures on a page. I see large sums of money spent but not wisely. I see poor direction, organizational chaos, and wasted resources that in most cases will not leave enrollees and communities much better off than they are today.

Regardless of the future stability and success of integrated health care systems, it is imperative that health care professionals understand the definition, the developmental process, and the factors that contribute to both success and failure of integrated health care systems. Professionals already in the health care field and students who are on their way there are the audience for this book. Some will make decisions about integration; others will be affected by those decisions. All will feel the impact.

The purpose of this book is threefold. The first goal is to educate. Senior and midlevel health care administrators, managers, and clinicians need to understand integrated health care in terms to which they can comfortably relate. In many organizations, a handful of key decision makers embark on a strategy of integration but do not communicate the message to others. People whose daily activities are directly affected by integration often lack a basic understanding of the concept. They have no context for their organization's activities and their own responsibilities. Education about integrated health care is also essential for students. At some point in their careers, they will work within an integrated setting or in collaboration with an integrated system. They need to understand their options and opportunities.

A second purpose of the book is to guide health care decision makers in their integration efforts. A principal theme is that thoughtful planning, appreciation for the evolutionary nature of integration, and attention to relationships are very important. Attention to proven success factors and common barriers can ease the way.

Finally, this book is for people outside the health care system who hear about and experience changes but do not understand what they are. Enrollees, suppliers, vendors, public and private payers, and regulatory bodies are all dealing with integrated health care, like it or not.

The book is divided into seven chapters and two appendices.

Chapter 1 provides a general definition of integrated health care systems. It describes multiple applications of the term integration: horizontal, vertical, functional, clinical, virtual, and visual.

Chapter 2 sets the stage. It describes the three factors in the external environment that stimulate the formation of integrated systems: market focus, reimbursement, and expectations for delivery and coordination of care.

Chapter 3 describes the general process of creating, maintaining, and continually fine-tuning integrated health care systems. It identifies three macro issues that systems repeatedly revisit (market, organization, and internal functions) and seven common growth stages (preliminary planning, system formation, assimilation, market moves, acceptance of the importance of systems, redesign, and community health and advocacy). The chapter also describes how macro issues and growth stages interact with one another.

Chapter 4 identifies and describes factors that contribute to but do not guarantee system success. These include philosophical commitment to system development, clarity of purpose and vision, physician involvement in key leadership roles, alignment of financial incentives and rewards, customer focus, information systems and technology that support system goals and operations, ongoing emphasis on quality improvement, and focus on creating value.

Chapter 5 describes barriers that surface at different points in time during systems evolution. These include failures to develop and communicate a vision of the end and interim states; identify target populations and desirable outcomes; plan for capital needs; anticipate potential legal barriers; address differences in philosophy and culture; take the time to build trust; identify important leadership characteristics and recruit/train talent; understand the importance of primary care; come to terms with governance; address inequities in resources, information, and benefits; clarify lines of authority; and manage the unique aspects of integrated systems.

Chapter 6 contains short cases that illustrate many of the points made in the first five chapters. No single system is a model for all aspects of system development, and the examples come from systems of different sizes, sponsorships, and geographic locations. They include large systems in mature managed care markets and smaller systems in places where managed care is less dominant. Urban and rural systems are included.

Chapter 7 is an in-depth case study of Duke University Medical Center & Health System in Durham, N.C., during its start-up phase from 1992 to 1996.

The appendix, by Eve T. Horwitz, addresses legal issues. The glossary defines terms as they relate to integrated delivery systems.

Colleagues throughout the country have been generous with their insights and suggestions. My thanks go to the following and to Rena Wethington, my staff assistant at Duke University Medical Center & Health System; Robert W. Anderson, MD; Daniel Barco, MD; Peter Boland, PhD; Lawton R. Burns, PhD; Jeanne Chamberlin; Allan Chrisman, MD; Dennis Clements, MD; Janis Curtis; William J. Donelan; Susan Epstein; Eve T. Horwitz; Arnold D. Kaluzny, PhD; Elizabeth J. Kramer; Peter Kussin, MD; Rex McCallum, MD; J. Lloyd Michener, MD; James J. Morris, MD; John H. Paat, MD; Andy Pasternack; Stephen Pollock, MD; Paul Rosenberg; Vicki Saito, Steven Sauter; Kevin C. Stone; Robert Taber, PhD; Margaret S. Veach; Samuel W. Warburton, MD; and Duncan Yaggy, PhD.

Durham, N.C.
April 1997

References

The Advisory Board Company. 1995. *Emerging from shadow: Resurgence to prosperity under managed care.* Washington, D.C.: The Advisory Board Company.

Findlay, S. 1996. Columbia/HCA wants to sing the blues. *Business and Health* 14 (1): 9 (January).

Kertesz, L. 1996. Aetna deal signals provider squeeze. *Modern Healthcare* 26 (15): 2, 3, 13 (8 April).

Kropko, M. R. 1996. Rite aid deal to be challenged. *The News and Observer*, 18 April, 9C.

Lessons from the break-up of a promising joint venture. 1996. *Health System Leader* 3 (2): 2–3 (March).

Lutz, S. 1996. Sowing the seeds of partnership between providers, managed care. *Modern Healthcare* 26 (15): 32–33 (8 April).

Much ado about mergers and acquisitions. 1996. *Business and Health* 14 (1): 9 (January).

News at deadline. 1996. *Modern Healthcare* 26 (2): 4 (8 January).

PacifiCare plans to acquire rival FHP, Inc. for $2 billion. 1996. *BNAs Managed Care Reporter* 2 (33): 786 (14 August).

Shriver, K. 1995. Study of networks up 69% in 1995. *Modern Healthcare* 25 (26): 26 (26 June).

Sokolov, J. 1996. Presentation at Private Sector Conference, 15 April, at Duke University Medical Center, Durham, N.C.

Yandell, L. 1997. Interview by author. Premier. Charlotte, N.C., 9 April.

1

"Integrated Health Care Systems": Definition and Applications

INTRODUCTION

When people talk about integration in health care, they do not always speak the same language. It is therefore important to begin with a general definition of integrated health care systems and to address different applications of the term *integration*. These include horizontal, vertical, functional, clinical, virtual, and visual.

WHAT IS AN INTEGRATED SYSTEM AND WHAT DOES IT DO?

Regardless of the unique organizational and operational characteristics of integrated health care systems, most of them aspire to meet five objectives. Described by Stephen Shortell and his colleagues in their 1996 longitudinal evaluation of 11 systems, these are market focus; provision of a continuum of care; reliance on information; alignment of financial incentives and organizational structures; and development and maintenance of ongoing efforts to improve quality (Shortell and others 1996).

Focuses on Meeting the Needs of Its Market

Integrated health care systems that are aware of and attentive to market needs develop, organize, provide, and sometimes finance the provision of health care services in response to the needs of both populations and individuals. When they assume financial risk, they become attentive to the needs of the populations for which they are responsible. They commit to keeping people and populations healthy by preventive care, provision of care to those who become ill, and restoration to good health.

Ideally, the process of market assessment begins with the identification of the geographic areas and/or populations for which a system will assume responsibility. Geographic coverage may be national, regional, or local. Enrollment targets generally drive geographic coverage, although in rural areas, geography may dictate enrollment. With respect to target populations, systems may include commercial and/or publicly insured groups.

Given the economics of health care, neither individuals nor populations are likely to purchase care directly from integrated systems. Purchasers such as private employers, purchasing groups, and public payers make decisions on behalf of the individuals and groups they represent.

Once systems are clear about geographic coverage and target populations, they can use existing and new information to develop baseline profiles of individuals and groups. They can respond to the data in two overlapping ways. To meet the needs of individual enrollees, they can provide, organize, and coordinate education, treatment, and follow-up. To meet group needs, they can develop education, prevention, and treatment that they expect will improve the overall health of specific population sectors.

Integrated systems' attention and readjustment to market needs occurs at many points in time during their evolution. The process is ongoing and not an activity with a distinct beginning and end. Most systems look hard at market factors during feasibility, after initial start-up, and during expansion (Jones and Mayerhofer 1994).

Although formal attention to the health and wellness of particular populations is relatively new to the health care delivery system, the concept of assessing and responding to community needs is a familiar one in the health care industry. Public health activities have taken this approach for many years. Health care organizations founded by religious groups have devoted a great deal of attention to identifying and meeting the needs of populations that might have difficulty accessing and/or paying for care. Public and private academic medical centers have a tradition of providing care to the less fortunate in society (For-profit conversions 1996). Managed health care plans that have assumed financial risk for the care of their members have experience with population-based care. More recent motivations for responding to community health needs are justification of tax status and response to antitrust concerns by regulatory agencies.

Provides Continuum of Care

To meet the needs of both populations and individuals, integrated health care systems can offer different levels of care in a variety of settings. As shown in figure 1-1, the continuum of care includes at least health education and wellness, primary care, acute care management, tertiary and quaternary care, supportive care (home care), subacute care, long-term care, rehabilitation, and skilled nursing care. The patient and family, not the sites at which the

FIGURE 1-1. Continuum of Care

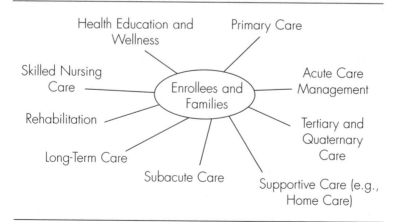

care is delivered, are central. The challenge for integrated health care systems is to go beyond the provision of care. They must also coordinate care in ways that meet the needs of patients, families, employers, and other payers.

Relies on Information

Integrated health care systems need information to understand the health needs of both populations and individuals. Information about health status, public health problems, historical utilization of health care, and the cost of care delivery helps them determine what care to provide and how to coordinate it.

Systems also need information so they can measure what they are doing. They need to look at the outcomes of their efforts, and to compare their own performance against an external baseline. They also need to look at performance trends over time to see if they are improving system deficiencies and shortcomings.

Accurate, comprehensive, patient-focused information can contribute to better quality of care that meets the standards of consumers, providers, payers, and regulators. When systems combine information that has been gathered at different sites of care, they have opportunities to develop profiles for individuals and groups, organize and modify the care they deliver, improve care management, and provide care within financial constraints.

Finally, systems can use information to establish and maintain accountability. Patients, payers, employers, employees, community groups, and external review bodies are all interested in what systems do, how they do it, how much money they spend, and what their outcomes are.

Aligns Financial and Organizational Objectives

The financing and delivery of health care in the United States is an unwieldy combination of private enterprise and public entitlement. The proliferation of different methods of reimbursement for care has created confusion for caregivers and payers. Conflicting financial incentives send mixed messages, and the confusion is often within a single organization. Organizational goals, like financial incentives, are not always consistent. Integrated health care systems aspire to realign both financial and organizational incentives so that their component parts are consistently motivated to provide, coordinate, and manage care.

Maintains Continuous Effort to Improve Quality of Care

Finally, integrated health care systems look for ways in which to impact and demonstrate improvement in the health care provided to individuals and populations. Different interest groups have varying perspectives on what needs to be improved; progressive systems are sensitive to the expectations of enrollees, providers, payers, and the community. Systems' attention to the improvement of care is ongoing throughout the entire process of system growth and evolution.

APPLICATIONS OF "INTEGRATED HEALTH CARE"

Different applications of the term *integration* are often used as if they were synonymous, confusing people both inside and outside the health care industry. A practical approach for understanding integration is to distinguish the different uses of the term: horizontal, vertical, clinical, functional, virtual, and visual (table 1-1).

Horizontal Integration

Horizontal integration within integrated health care systems applies to lateral relationships among like entities. If, for example, a system includes multiple hospitals, physicians, ambulatory sites, home care, and other components, horizontal integration means the formal and informal structural and working relationships between and among the entities in each category.

Examples of integration of like entities are abundant. They apply to hospitals, physicians, health plans, insurers, and suppliers. In the hospital field, an example of integration among acute hospitals is Sun-Health Alliance. Between 1969 and 1994, hospitals in 15 southern states from Maryland to Texas came together as an alliance to pursue group activities that would enhance the success of each participant. Members retained separate corporate identities but benefited from

TABLE 1-1. Applications of Term "Integrated Health Care"

Type	Definition	Comment
Horizontal	Lateral relationships among like entities Often stepping-stone to vertical integration	Important issue: number of operating units providing same service
Vertical	Coordinating, linking, or incorporating within a single organization activities or entities at different stages of the production and delivery of patient care	Common methods: mergers, alliances, PHOs
Functional	Coordination of key support functions and activities across operating units	Examples: human resources, support services, culture, strategic planning, quality assurance, marketing, information systems, financial management
Clinical	Continuity of care; coordination of care; disease management; good caregiver communication; smooth transfer of patient information and records; elimination of duplication; efficient use and management of resources	Techniques: clinical protocols; care management; uniform and accessible medical records; collection and use of clinical outcomes data; clinical program/facility planning; shared clinical support services; and service lines
Virtual	Emphasis on relationships, not asset ownership, as means for collaboration among system components	Less tangible but more important than ownership. Can co-exist with asset owernship.
Visual	Delivery of health care and linkage of information in ways that look like a single system	Market's way of evaluating systems

opportunities available to the collective body. In 1995, SunHealth reaffirmed its commitment to the alliance type of integration. Moving beyond the southeast region, it merged with a much larger alliance, AmHS/Premier, to form the new Premier (Rethmeier 1996).

Physicians, like hospitals, may integrate with one another to survive and thrive. Common ways in which physicians integrate are group practices, management service organizations (MSOs), and independent practice associations (IPAs). Sometimes, but not always, physician-only integration precedes physician integration with other entities. For example, when physicians and hospitals decide to form physician-hospital organizations (PHOs), physicians who plan to join the PHO may strengthen the physician-only part of the organization by first forming an IPA.

Integration among like entities is not restricted to health care providers. Managed health care plans and insurance companies often look for ways to attract greater market share. Mergers with other plans and insurers may facilitate expansion of product offerings and/or appeal to larger geographic areas.

Horizontal integration has potential advantages, including economies of scale, access to scarce resources, and collective bargaining power (Zuckerman, Kaluzny, and Ricketts 1995). If these positive outcomes are realized within particular components of a system, the entire system—that is, the total enterprise—may have a better chance of achieving its strategic goals. For example, in a system that includes 10 acute hospitals with duplication of services, the hospitals may collaborate in service line planning. Stronger service lines can benefit the entire system.

Horizontal integration, especially among hospitals, can be a stepping-stone to vertical integration among unlike entities and/or integration of health care delivery and financing. For example:

- Advocate Health Care is the result of a full asset merger between two previously existing systems, Lutheran General Health System and Evangelical Health System in Park Ridge, Ill., which brought together two successful systems. Each had already undergone some degree of horizontal and vertical integration (Risk and Francis 1994).
- The North Shore Medical Center in Salem, Mass., accomplished significant horizontal integration among local hospitals and vertical integration between those hospitals and local physicians before and after becoming part of the larger Partners HealthCare System.

■ Partners HealthCare System in eastern Massachusetts regards its approach to horizontal integration among physicians as an important component of its total vertical system strategy. Partners created a separate organization, Partners Community HealthCare, Inc. (PCHI), to integrate 850 to 900 practicing physicians. Initially PCHI expected that relationships with all these physicians would be parallel. Over time, however, it became clear that physicians in different practice settings and different communities had different needs, and that diversity, not similarity in structure, would be more likely to achieve horizontal physician integration. Some physicians sold their practices to PCHI. Others use PCHI as an MSO. Still others prefer contractual arrangements. From a system perspective, the different physician arrangements do not hinder the development of standardized medical management and quality of care (Zane 1996).

When horizontal integration occurs, systems must determine the number of operating units that will provide the same service. For example, how many beds at various levels? How many physicians in different specialties? How much home care capacity? Technically, an integrated system that has identified the population for which it will assume responsibility can size its delivery system to meet that population's needs, taking into consideration special issues such as access, population mix, and public health factors. Figure 1-2 shows a worksheet for determining system capacity.

In a political world, however, depth of integration in health care systems is not scientific, especially when systems begin. Many systems tolerate initial excess capacity in order to link organizations that will accelerate enrollment growth. More important, many new integrated systems include a cash-rich organization that provides financial support above and beyond that of other system components. If that particular organization is overbedded, overstaffed, or oversized in some other way, the entire system may delay addressing its capacity issue until the political climate is right for downsizing this component.

Of all the issues related to systems' size, one stands out: primary care capacity. Many systems have realized that an adequate supply of primary care providers and other caregivers who are physically located in places that are convenient to existing and potential members has the greatest impact. If people cannot select primary care providers, access to the rest of the system, regardless of size, will be difficult.

FIGURE 1-2. Worksheet for Determining System Capacity in Horizontal Integration

Instructions: Determine basic system capacity and use special factors to make modifications.				
Enrollment Level				
Component	Target Ratio/100 Members	Actual Ratio/100 Members	Special Factors	Recommended Adjustment Needed
Health Education and Wellness				
Primary Care				
Acute Care Management				
Tertiary and Quaternary Care				
Supportive Care (Home Care)				
Subacute Care				
Long-Term Care				
Rehabilitation				
Skilled Nursing Care				
Special factors that might modify basic system capacity: • Access Issues • Population Mix • Public Health Information				

Vertical Integration

Integration is not always among like organizations that produce the same product. As the concept of providing a continuum of care gains popularity, organizations that have historically provided one type of care have joined with or contracted with organizations that provide other kinds of care.

A good definition of vertical integration comes from industry: "linking the production functions of individual organizations that either precede or follow another organization's core business operations within the boundaries of a new organization" (Thompson 1967). In health care, vertical integration means "coordinating, linking, or incorporating within a single organization activities or entities at different stages of a production process . . . i.e., producing and delivering patient care" (Conrad and Dowling 1990).

Vertical integration can link sites where care is delivered with patients, enrollees, and purchasers. It also can link the health care delivery system with suppliers and producers. If vertical integration is very aggressive, there is a link between health care delivery and financing.

The linkage of health care delivery and financing into "integrated health organizations," or IHOs, is controversial (Burns and Thorpe 1995). There are strong opinions but no consensus on the wisdom of combining the two (case 6-7). Historically, some of the most reputable HMOs in the country have successfully linked health care delivery and financing. Kaiser and the Fallon Community Health Plan are examples. In response to changes in the marketplace, both have reexamined their strategies. For example, the Fallon Healthcare System (case 6-1), of which the Fallon Community Health Plan is a part, believes that at times its own health plan limits its future growth (Podbielski 1996).

Newer systems as well as older ones like Kaiser and Fallon have reevaluated the wisdom of combining health care delivery and financing under common ownership. For example, Graduate Health System in Philadelphia sold its HMO and other for-profit subsidiaries to Health Systems International (HSI) in an attempt to increase market share and access to capital (Cramer and Kmetz 1995). Within a year, Graduate began discussions with the larger Allegheny Health, Education, and Research Foundation (Pallarito 1996).

Integrated systems that believe both health care delivery and financing should be combined within a single system take different approaches to the balance of the two. The Allina Health System in Minnesota was formed in July 1994 with the merger of two successful organizations, an IHO (HealthSpan) and a health plan (Medica). Allina's unique co-CEO arrangement reflects the importance given to both delivery system and health plan components of the enterprise (Pacesetters 1995).

Other systems that have integrated both health care delivery and financing are more comfortable with delivery system domination. The Henry Ford Health System in Michigan includes hospitals, physicians, alternative care, and health plans offered through the Alliance Health and Life Insurance Company (AHLIC). Available health plan options include an HMO, preferred provider organization (PPO), and

▪ SIDEBAR

Alliances

Strategic alliances allow different organizations to pool resources, ally to exploit opportunities, and/or link systems in partnership arrangements (Kanter and Stein 1993). They are common in industry, both inside and outside the health care field. At times alliances have allowed pursuit of activities that might be difficult to do alone. They can also be passive, rather than active, and provide participants with an opportunity for mutual learning.

Alliances are built on relationships. They are less formalized than joint ventures, contracts, mergers, and acquisitions. However, once formed, they require ongoing management to survive; this point is often forgotten. A major challenge is that management of partners is not the same as management of subordinates. Successful leadership in alliances requires skill in creating good linkages among organizations and in communicating within and between organizations.

Not all alliances work. Reasons for failure include imbalances in resources, information, and benefits; miscommunication; misplaced trust; conflicting loyalties; and undermanagement. When alliances are dependent on visionary individuals, there is a risk that infrastructure and clear common purpose will never become institutionalized (Stein 1995; Zuckerman, Kaluzny, and Ricketts 1995).

Despite the pitfalls, some very good health care alliances have been in place for many years. They have met member needs over time and have been able to change when necessary. Examples are described in case 6-2.

▪ SIDEBAR

Physician-Hospital Organizations

Health care organizations may use PHOs to achieve vertical integration. The entities that come together are (1) physicians in diverse practice settings and disciplines and (2) hospitals. Two common reasons that PHOs form are to share administrative services and costs and to improve bargaining power with payers. From the physicians' vantage point, other potential advantages can include increased administrative expertise, reduced administrative overhead, and access to capital. From the hospitals' perspective, among the potential benefits are increased physician loyalty, access to covered lives, and solidification of a primary care and ambulatory care base.

In a report on PHOs published in February 1995, Ernst & Young summarized the results of a survey of 189 organizations. Results revealed much to justify the conclusion that "PHOs have much potential to serve many roles," but "many are not yet adequately prepared to pursue them" (Ernst & Young 1995). Most PHOs are young organizations; nearly 75 percent studied were less than one year old. Although some had contracts for covered lives, most did not have many. PHOs were operationally immature with respect to staffing levels and experience. They had difficulty working out relationships between physicians and hospitals and between primary care and specialist physicians.

Aside from operational immaturity, a problem that time can correct, certain PHO arrangements have the potential to negatively impact the tax-exempt status of not-for-profit hospitals. Even within the PHO movement, there is skepticism regarding the long-term survival of stand-alone PHOs (Expansion 1995). State and federal regulation is a major unresolved issue. The frequency of government pronouncements at both levels contributes to PHOs' vulnerability. The National Association of Insurance Commissioners and the HMO industry have expressed concern about the lack of regulation of PHOs, particularly those that are capitated for covered lives and act like insurance companies (Burns 1995; Expansion 1995). In a September 1995 ruling, the U.S. Justice Department ruled that physicians in PHOs must take on financial risk if they expect to compete with HMOs and other managed care organizations (A major move 1995).

Nonetheless, some PHOs have overcome some of the obstacles, met current needs of physicians and hospitals, and also accepted the reality that they may be transitional strategies. One example is North

Shore Health System, the PHO developed by the North Shore Medical Center in Salem, Mass. (Montague 1995). The organization was formed when an unsuccessful hospital merger threatened to destroy the futures of a loyal cadre of physicians. Physician leadership is particularly strong and has influenced both the local system and the regional system of which it is a part. North Shore has the ability to accept capitation, pay claims, and assume delegated responsibility for utilization management (case 6-12).

---

point-of-service plan (POS). Although AHLIC is important, it has not precluded the development of contractual relationships with many other health plans (Nighswander 1994). Sisters of Providence in Portland, Ore., has joined multiple managed care products under the umbrella of Sisters of Providence Health Plans (Shortell and others 1996). Finally, Duke University Medical Center & Health System in Durham, N.C., has a joint venture with a major insurer, but has also continued to contract with many other managed health care plans (see chapter 7).

Some of the advantages of vertical integration are similar to those that can be achieved from horizontal integration: economies of scale and increased operating efficiency. However, those concerning alignment of financing and governance incentives and provision of continuity of care are different.

Three methods to achieve vertical integration are mergers, alliances, and PHOs. Although formal mergers may appear to be the preferred strategy for integration because the result is immediately visible, merged organizations often ignore the importance of building relationships. On the other hand, alliances depend on relationships—in fact, some have existed for more than 20 years (Dowling 1995). PHOs are a more recent phenomenon. To date they have shown more promise than performance (Ernst & Young 1995).

Functional Integration

Systems' decisions about market area, structure, and legal form are just the tip of the iceberg. Still to come are two challenging aspects of integration: functional and clinical integration. Both must be planned, implemented, monitored, and continuously fine-tuned.

Shortell and his colleagues define functional integration as "the extent to which key support functions and activities . . . are coordinated across operating units so as to add the greatest overall value to the system" (Shortell and others 1996). Examples of these functions and activities are human resources, support services, culture, strategic planning, quality assurance, marketing, information systems, and financial management (both resource allocation and operating policies).

Functional integration does not imply that all activities should be centralized and/or standardized. The important question is, "Does the strategy meet system goals?" Functional integration also does not imply that all functions and activities must be reorganized simultaneously. There is often a definite logic to addressing some functions before others. For example, strategic planning, which results in consensus on organizational mission and goals and establishes a model for good communication throughout the system, should begin as early as possible. It can lay a strong foundation for other activities. As described in chapters 4 and 5, however, many systems neglect the importance of early systemwide planning, only to find themselves on an accelerated course to nowhere because other activities are dependent on a coherent plan.

Functional integration is challenging. When it works well, factors that often contribute to its success are thoughtful strategic planning, skilled leadership, buy-in by all operating units, attention to the creation of a unified culture, use of continuous quality improvement/total quality management (CQI/TQM) techniques, early attention to information systems and technology, relationship of individual financial incentives to system performance, and creation of a methodology for system self-monitoring.

When functional integration fails, there are also common causes. One common obstacle is limited understanding of system vision. When only the "privileged few" know where the system is headed, system development is less likely to progress smoothly than it is when the entire organization is clear on the long-term goals and planned sequence of steps. A second barrier to functional integration is difficulty in knowing when to centralize and standardize; there are relatively few models to examine, and methods for building integrated systems are not found in textbooks. A third obstacle is lack of commitment among operating units. Often one or more hospitals with more money and influence than other system components dominate discussions and undermine the cooperative spirit.

Lack of capable personnel is yet another problem; relatively few leaders in the health care field have had the breadth of experience needed to build and operate integrated systems. Finally, underestimating the urgency of addressing inequities can become an underlying deterrent to system progress. For example, if employees of different organizations within the same system are compensated according to different pay scales and financial incentives, the inequity may affect their commitment to making the system work.

Baylor Health Care System in Dallas/Fort Worth, Tex., and Advocate Health Care in Illinois have taken functional integration seriously and made good progress (Shortell and others 1996). An overview of those systems is shown in case 6-3.

Clinical Integration

One of the respondents in Shortell's study stated frankly, "Clinical integration is like pornography. Everyone recognizes it when they see it" (Shortell and others 1996). Clinical integration includes continuity of care, coordination of care, disease management, good communication among caregivers, smooth transfer of information and patient records, elimination of duplicate testing and procedures, and efficient use and management of resources. The ultimate goal of clinical integration is to "mass customize"—that is, create a method for delivering and measuring care that has common efficiencies but meets individual needs (Kotha 1995).

The importance of clinical integration is clear. Shortell and his colleagues believe it is the most important aspect of integration. Douglas A. Conrad, of the University of Washington Department of Health Services, has commented, "administrative and organizational-managerial integration is a necessary complement to the clinical integration of patient care, but it is the latter that is crucial to achieve a viable vertically integrated regional health system" (Conrad 1993). Frank D. Kittredge of The Bristol Group in Boston says, "to be truly successful in managing the care of the large population it seeks to serve, an integrated delivery system must establish as its long-term goals the measurable improvement of the outcomes of care and experience of the patients it serves and the ability to successfully provide health care for a market price. . . . What's required to achieve this goal is the clinical integration of the system" (Kittredge 1996). It is interesting that, in September 1996, the Justice Department and Federal Trade Commission jointly issued revisions of antitrust guidelines for provider-sponsored organizations, identifying clinical integration as justification for receiving rule of reason treatment (Revised guidelines 1996).

Although they are not guarantees, some of the techniques that help systems achieve clinical integration are clinical protocols; care management programs; uniform and accessible medical records; collection and use of clinical outcomes data; planning of clinical programs and facilities; shared clinical support services; and shared clinical service lines.

Common barriers to the achievement of clinical integration fall into four broad categories: strategic, structural, cultural, and technical (Shortell and others 1996). Their impact varies depending upon the market stage in which the system functions.

Stage 1 markets are relatively unstructured; patients have maximum access to care, and there is little pressure on providers to reduce the cost of care. Stage 2 markets can be described as "loose cost." In both stage 1 and 2 markets, hospitals probably dominate the market and have not yet accepted the reality that they are a revenue center of a larger system, not the center of the universe. Physicians are unlikely to be organized into groups. There is minimal hospital/physician coordination. In general, there is little external pressure to change and minimal internal interest in clinical integration.

In stage 3 (consolidated advanced cost) and stage 4 (strict managed care) markets, other barriers to clinical integration arise. They are geography; failure to develop a plan/strategy for clinical integration; failure to align budgeting, performance appraisal, and reward systems; fear of job loss; inadequate information systems; and lack of population-based planning. Details on some of the barriers to clinical integration follow.

Geography can inhibit clinical integration if operating units are located so far apart that they cannot establish shared clinical service lines, staffing, and other support services (Scott 1996). Some systems address the geographic barrier by regionalizing their management. Examples are Advocate Health Care in Illinois; Sisters of Providence in Oregon (Kaluzny 1994); and Kaiser. In 1996, Kaiser Foundation Health Plan and Hospitals created six divisions, each composed of local markets, so that division leaders could be more responsive to local business planning and growth (Kertesz 1996).

Ideally, clinical integration involves three steps: (1) determination of vision and assessment of readiness; (2) development of strategy and planning; and (3) implementation and measurement

(Gorvine and Kittredge 1997). Many systems fail to address all three components. They may permit or actively encourage the development of multiple efforts that are unrelated to one another and/or to an overall system strategy. For example, academic medical centers often struggle with a culture that encourages initiative and entrepreneurial behavior. Clinical integration may conflict with individually sponsored projects. In the public sector, the Veterans Administration vision from Washington may ignore wide fluctuations in regional and local readiness.

Failure to align budgeting, performance appraisal, and reward systems sends a confusing message to clinicians and administrative staff and obstructs clinical integration. Senior-level leaders may have different financial incentives from midlevel managers, who must actualize the plans.

Fear of job loss is another barrier to clinical integration. Numbers of clinicians have changed from inpatient to outpatient practice and participated in restructuring the delivery of clinical care, only to find that they have restructured themselves out of their jobs or been transferred within the system. Employees whose positions are not eliminated may find that job realignment and restructuring are stressful.

Inadequacy of information systems obviously impacts ability to achieve clinical integration. When patient-specific information cannot cross organizational lines—that is, inpatient/outpatient or acute/nonacute care—clinicians and administrators do not have the information that might help them make meaningful changes and measure the results. Duplication of effort is not eliminated.

Finally, delayed population-based planning inhibits clinical integration. Although logic suggests that needs assessment should precede program development, the latter more often comes first. If a system addresses population-based planning last, it may not tailor the scope and delivery of services to the populations for which it is responsible.

In clinical integration, as in functional, the existence of formidable barriers does not mean that no systems succeed (Shortell and others 1996). For example, Mercy Health Services in Michigan has developed a clinical integration plan. Fairview Hospital and Healthcare Services in Minnesota has done sophisticated population-based planning and created a department of community health.

Structural initiatives that contribute to success in clinical integration include alignment of internal financial incentives, development of a group practice or grouplike structure, creation of a unit that is responsible for clinical effectiveness and outcomes support (for example, Henry Ford Health System in Michigan and Advocate Health Care in Illinois), and patient care restructuring (such as Sentara in Virginia).

Cultural factors that facilitate clinical integration include commitment to the CQI/TQM process (for example, Henry Ford Health System, Sentara, and Advocate Health Care), retraining workers (Sharp in California), and development of formal training for physician leadership (Henry Ford Health System).

Information systems, reengineering, and joint professional education are technical factors that can facilitate clinical integration.

Virtual Integration

There are two major misconceptions about integrated health care delivery and financing systems:

- Full asset mergers and accumulation of bricks and mortar pave the road to success.
- Ownership guarantees "value."

Private industry knows many things that the health care field stubbornly ignores, despite repeated warnings by a handful of respected health care leaders. According to Jeff Goldsmith of Health Futures, Inc., "After surveying the literature and reflecting on fourteen years of consulting experience working with systems, I find it stunning how little hard evidence of economic advantage or market share has accrued from system development in health care." He continues, "The core flaw in the integration movement in heathcare is the use of an obsolete 19th-century asset-based model of integration, in which accumulation of assets in a conglomerate style is assumed by itself to confer meaningful economic advantage" (Goldsmith 1994). Shortell has suggested that belief in the inevitability of systems by the people who are making them is what propels them. He believes their value is vague. Finally, in its 1996 survey of more than 200 integrated delivery and financing systems, Ernst & Young noted that many systems lacked infrastructure, management commitment, and strategic planning (Japsen 1996).

Goldsmith and other experts put more faith in virtual integration, wherein organizations behave as if they are a part of a larger organization. They believe that relationships count more than structures, and that structures do not guarantee collaboration. One example of virtual integration that bears watching over time is the Alliance Network in Oregon that links Legacy Health System's hospital and specialty system with three medical clinics collectively called Northwest Physician Alliance and with Blue Cross and Blue Shield of Oregon.

Visual Integration

After all is said and done, if the structure, relationships, and inner workings of integrated health care systems do not deliver care to consumers, link information, and meet the needs of consumers and providers in ways that *look like a single system,* all the accomplishments along the way are meaningless.

One *Fortune* 500 company suggests that, as a buyer, it is not interested in purchasing from a system that cannot get its act together. Even when the system price is lower than a nonsystem price might be, if that system's internal workings do not function properly, the experience of the enrollees who receive care may not be a good one.

Shortell believes that the jury on integrated health care is still out. The "value" of integration has not yet been proven (Shortell and others 1996).

References

Burns, J. 1995. Insurance commissioners deserve respect: Industry's focus on solvency raises questions for plan sponsors. *Managed Healthcare* 5 (12): 30 (December).

Burns, L. R., and D. P. Thorpe. 1995. Managed care and integrated health care. *Health Care Management: State of the Art Reviews* 2 (1): 101–108 (October).

Conrad, D. A. 1993. Coordinating patient care services in regional health systems: The challenge of clinical integration. *Journal of the Foundation of the ACHE* 38 (4): 491–507 (winter).

Conrad, D. A., and W. L. Dowling. 1990. Vertical integration in health services: Theory and managerial implications. *Health Care Management Review* 15 (4): 9–22 (fall).

Cramer, H., and J. Kmetz. 1995. Interview by author. Graduate Health System, Philadelphia, 19 September.

Dowling, W. L. 1995. Strategic alliances as a structure for integrated delivery systems. In *Partners for the dance: Forming strategic alliances in health care,* edited by A. D. Kaluzny, H. S. Zuckerman, and T. C. Ricketts. Ann Arbor: Health Administration Press.

Ernst & Young LLP. 1995. *Physician-hospital organization profile.* Washington, D.C.: Ernst & Young LLP.

Expansion is critical for survival of your PHO. 1995. *Hospital Integrated Care Report* 3 (4): 47–48 (April).

For-profit conversions must come with a commitment to community. 1996. *Modern Healthcare* 26 (16): 40 (15 April).

Goldsmith, J. C. 1994. The illusive logic of integration. *Healthcare Forum Journal* 37 (5): 26–31 (September/October).

Gorvine, B., and F. D. Kittredge. 1997. Clinical integration: Steps you must take to achieve it. *The Bristol Review.* February.

Japsen, B. 1996. Survey: Integrated systems pale next to HMOs. *Modern Healthcare* 26 (32): 10 (5 August).

Jones, W. J., and J. J. Mayerhofer. 1994. Regional health care systems: Implications for health care reform. *Managed Care Quarterly* 2 (1): 31–44 (winter).

Kaluzny, A. D. 1994. Centralization and decentralization in a vertically integrated system: The XYZ hospital corporation. In *Strategic alignment: Managing integrated health systems,* edited by D. A. Conrad and G. A. Hoare. Ann Arbor: AUPHA Press/Health Administration Press.

Kanter, R. M., and B. A. Stein. 1993. *Strategic alliances: Some lessons from experience.* Cambridge, Mass.: Goodmeasure, Inc.

Kertesz, L. 1996. Changing structure. *Modern Healthcare* 26 (37): 14 (9 September).

Kittredge, F. D. 1996. What is clinical integration and why is it so important? *The Bristol Review*. October.

Kotha, S. 1995. Mass customization: Implementing the emerging paradigm for competitive advantage. *Strategic Management Journal* 16:21–42 (summer).

A major move toward regulating PHOs. 1995. *Business and Health* 13 (10): 9 (October).

Montague, J. 1995. When the smoke clears. *Hospitals and Health Networks* 69 (3): 65–68 (5 February).

Nighswander, A. 1994. *Integrated health care delivery: A blueprint for action*. St. Paul: InterStudy Publications.

Pacesetters. 1995. Supplement to *Hospitals and Health Networks*. November.

Pallarito, K. 1996. Allegheny adds to Philadelphia ranks. *Modern Healthcare* 26 (33):10 (12 August).

Podbielski, J. 1996. Interview by author. Fallon Clinic, Inc., Worcester, Mass., 15 July.

Rethmeier, K. 1996. Interview by author. Premier, Charlotte, N.C., 13 June.

Revised guidelines will boost PSO growth, but unlikely to impact HMOs analysts say. 1996. *BNAs Managed Care Reporter* 2 (37): 884–886 (18 September).

Risk, R. R., and C. P. Francis. 1994. Transforming a hospital facility company into an integrated medical care organization. *Managed Care Quarterly* 2 (4): 12–23 (fall).

Scott, K. Integrating clinical service lines. 1996. *Health System Leader* 3 (2): 4–11 (March).

Shortell, S. M., R. R. Gillies, D. A. Anderson, K. M. Erickson, and J. B. Mitchell. 1996. *Remaking health care in America: Building organized delivery systems*. San Francisco: Jossey-Bass.

Stein, B. A. 1995. Strategic alliances: Some lessons from experience. In *Partners for the dance: Forming strategic alliances in health care,* edited by A. D. Kaluzny, H. S. Zuckerman, and T. C. Ricketts. Ann Arbor: Health Administration Press.

Thompson, J. D. 1967. *Organizations in action.* New York: McGraw-Hill.

Zane, E. 1996. Interview by author. Partners HealthCare System, Inc., Boston, 18 April.

Zuckerman, H. S., A. D. Kaluzny, and T. C. Ricketts. 1995. Strategic alliances: A worldwide phenomenon comes to health care. In *Partners for the dance: Forming strategic alliances in health care,* edited by A. D. Kaluzny, H. S. Zuckerman, and T. C. Ricketts. Ann Arbor: Health Administration Press.

2

External Environment: Impact on Systems Formation

INTRODUCTION

Although a proportion of health care executives and physicians engage in the development of integrated health care delivery/ financing systems because everyone else is doing it, most systems originate in response to events in the external environment. This chapter describes three aspects of the external environment that stimulate systems formation: market forces, reimbursement, and expectations for delivery and coordination of care (Satinsky 1995a and 1995b).

These three factors interact differently in different settings. However, in general they stimulate progression from an "unmanaged" to a "mature managed care" market as shown in table 2-1 (Shortell and others 1996). Although mature managed care markets receive much national attention, most localities in the United States fall somewhere in the middle. Realistically, they may never make it to maturity.

TABLE 2-1.   Suggested Level of Delivery System Integration Activity by Market Stage

Stage 1 Unstructured "access" market	Stage 2 "Loose cost" market	Stage 3 Consolidated "advanced cost" market	Stage 4 Strict managed care "value" market
• Acquire the pieces	• Expand functional integration efforts	• Expand physician-system integration efforts	• Expand clinical integration efforts
• Build functional integration	• Accelerate cost-reduction efforts	• Expand risk-based contracting	• Consolidate relationships with insurance partners
• Reduce costs	• Accelerate bed-reduction efforts	• Explore relationships with insurance partners	• Use outcomes data for external accountability and internal quality improvement
• Question the decentralization of capital to operating units	• Develop primary care physician network capacity	• Initiate clinical integration efforts	
• Look for physician and other partners	• Develop other parts of the continuum of care, e.g., home care	• Emphasize disease prevention and health promotion	• Expand population-based planning efforts
• Question acute inpatient focus	• Begin physician-system integration efforts	• Establish new management and governance structures	• Forge stronger partnerships with public health, community, and social service agencies
	• Begin to consolidate capital development		• Take greater responsibility for community health status and well being

Source: Shortell, S. M., R. R. Gillies, D. A. Anderson, K. M. Erickson, and J. B. Mitchell. 1996. *Remaking healthcare: Building organized delivery systems.* San Francisco: Jossey-Bass Publishers.

MARKET FORCES

Market characteristics that distinguish mature managed care environments from those that are less well developed are systems competition, focus on cost and quality, and prevalence of managed care coverage with leverage by a few strong health plans. In mature markets, integrated health care systems, not the separate components of which they are made, compete. Generally three to five large systems dominate. Health plans and employers develop strategies to contain health care costs while simultaneously ensuring provision of high-quality care. Also, 40 percent or more of people in both commercial and public sector markets are covered by managed care, and a few dominant HMOs are able to steer large numbers of enrollees from one system to another.

Minneapolis is a mature managed care market. Even in its maturity, however, it will continue to evolve. In late 1991, four major health systems controlled 70 percent of the hospital beds in the metropolitan area. Two of these systems, Health One and Life-Span, then merged to become HealthSpan. The Group Health and MedCenters HMOs then formed HealthPartners; that new entity became the holding company and joint manager for both plans.

Compared with those in the rest of the country, Minneapolis employers, like health systems and plans, were aggressive. Responding to President Clinton's proposed health alliance structure, a group of large employers solicited bids to form a competitive health plan. Four health care organizations formed the Institute for Clinical Systems Integration to focus on quality management, and HealthPartners, the Mayo Clinic, and Park Nicollet came together as major providers. Over time, the boundary between health care purchasers and health care delivery has blurred.

Boston exemplifies a metropolitan market that is rapidly moving toward maturity but is less developed than Minneapolis. Prior to 1994, competition in the health care market had been between like entities. Hospitals had competed with other hospitals, physicians had competed with their colleagues, and up to 20 managed care plans had competed with one another for market share.

However, market pressure by health plans and by private and public employers triggered a different response in the provider community. Providers initiated the formation of health care systems, and major academic medical centers assumed central roles. The Massachusetts General Hospital and Brigham and Women's Hospital, two Harvard Medical School teaching hospitals, came together and guided the creation of Partners HealthCare System, Inc. (Boston system 1996). Two other provider-initiated systems competed with Partners: provider-initiated CareGroup (formerly Pathway Health Network) and the Lahey-Hitchcock Clinic (Banks 1995). Partners and CareGroup contracted with but were not corporately linked with insurance partners. At the time, the Dartmouth-Hitchcock Medical Center contracted with the Matthew Thornton Health Plan, which has since been purchased by Harvard Pilgrim (Morrissey 1995).

Health Plans as a Way to Control Costs

Health care purchasers (health plans and employers) use many techniques to control health care costs while maintaining quality. Health plan strategies include but are not limited to market dominance through product diversification, benefit design, health plan consolidation, selective contracting, and demonstration of value.

Market Dominance through Product Diversification
To dominate the market, health plans diversify products. The more options they offer, the more able they are to meet diverse needs of private and public payers. Products that are commonly offered are staff and IPA model HMOs, PPOs, POS plans, indemnity insurance, and numerous combinations of these.

Another product diversification strategy is the linkage of workers' compensation insurance to health insurance. For example, CIGNA developed a system of bonuses and penalties designed to capture workers' comp business on a nationwide basis. Healthsource entered into workers' comp through alliances—for example, the Health Care Manager of New England in Massachusetts and Liberty Mutual Insurance Company in New Hampshire (Carriers 1996). A corporate survey of 241 companies conducted in 1996 by Watson-Wyatt Worldwide revealed that companies with managed disability programs were experiencing only half the costs of those with traditional approaches to disability (Integrated disability 1996).

Benefit Design   Benefit design is another way in which health plans distinguish themselves from competitors. Variations in covered services, referral requirements, premiums, and out-of-pocket costs can encourage payers to select a particular plan. For example, in late

1996, Oxford Health Plans became the first HMO in the country to offer its members access to a credentialed network of holistic practitioners. Commercial groups that select that option will pay a supplement to their HMO or POS coverage (Oxford 1996). Allina Health System in Minnesota also expressed interest in covering alternative health care therapies, pending results from a forthcoming study (Allina 1996).

Health Plan Consolidation   Some health plans decide that consolidation with other plans will increase market share and leverage with providers, improve access to capital, and ultimately facilitate growth. In fact, industry analysts predicted in 1996 that within the next decade, 90 percent of the HMO market would consolidate into 25 organizations that were local, regional, and national in origin (Merging 1996).

Health plan consolidation has occurred on different scales. Harvard Community Health Plan began as a Boston staff model plan. Acquisitions of group model plans in Massachusetts and Rhode Island enabled the Harvard Community Health Plan to diversify its product offerings and expand geographically. The plan's 1995 merger with a large IPA-type plan created even more opportunity for growth (Pham 1996). By April 1996, the consolidated Harvard Pilgrim Plan afforded 1.1 million subscribers access to 16,000 physicians. Within a few months, the new plan announced its intent to acquire New Hampshire's Matthew Thornton Health Plan, adding an additional 139,000 members (Harvard Pilgrim 1997).

At the state level, California has experienced major health plan consolidation. Although 1995 figures showed competition among more than 30 HMOs, consolidation of some of the largest plans with national presence created an enrollment-based three-tiered market of plans. At the top level were the giants, most of which had a national presence. These very large plans accounted for 85 percent of health plan enrollment. Plans in the middle and lower tiers were in different positions. The second tier accounted for only 10 percent of enrollment, and the lower tier had less than 5 percent. Over time, it is possible that competition will force even more consolidation in the two lower tiers (Cochrane 1996).

On a national level, there are many examples of health plan consolidation: Aetna/US Healthcare; Metropolitan and Travelers; MetraHealth and United Healthcare Corporation; and CIGNA Corp. and Healthsource, Inc.

Selective Contracting Another health plan strategy in mature managed care markets is selective contracting. In less-developed markets, both health plans and providers contract with many parties. However, over time, they may realize that fewer and more collaborative relationships might increase cost savings and mature into partnership arrangements. But selective contracting does not always go smoothly. Many states have passed "any willing provider" laws that require plans to contract with all providers who accept a certain level of reimbursement. These laws have been obstacles to selective contracting.

Demonstration of Health Plan Value Finally, health plans in mature markets have demonstrated "value" by measuring and distributing information on their clinical and operational performance. Recent efforts to demonstrate "accountability" differ from earlier efforts to become federally qualified and from standards formerly promulgated by industry organizations such as the former American Association of Preferred Provider Organizations. The new focus is on *consumer satisfaction.*

For example, in 1994, Kaiser's northern California region demonstrated its quality by generating a "report card" (Kenkel 1994). Kaiser defined quality as service delivery, not clinical outcomes, and measured seven areas: childhood health, maternal care, cardiovascular disease, cancer, common surgical procedures, other adult health, and mental health and substance abuse. It also examined member satisfaction with medical care, experience of care, access, and service.

The Advisory Board Company has suggested a broader set of indicators for self-evaluation and demonstration of value, including the following:

- Access measures showing enrollee ease in accessing the system
- Appropriateness measures comparing actual care rendered with expectations of care
- Service quality measures showing enrollee perceptions of the care received
- Encounter outcomes from an enrollee perspective
- Disease management measures showing the effectiveness of treating a disease in its entirety across the continuum of care
- Prevention measures showing the frequency and effectiveness of preventive care

■ Enrollee health status measures demonstrating the ability of the plan to maintain the health of the population for which it is responsible (Advisory Board Company 1994)

Within the past few years, health plans have increasingly sought recognition of their value from both the National Committee for Quality Assurance (NCQA) and the Joint Commission on Accreditation of Healthcare Organizations. NCQA was founded in 1990 as a not-for-profit organization. Its mission is to define quality, develop ways to measure it, and share that information with purchasers and the public. Since 1994, NCQA health plan accreditation status has been available to the public. Large employers such as AT&T, PepsiCo, US Airways, and Procter and Gamble consider only NCQA-accredited plans. Accreditation is difficult to achieve; only 42 percent of plans evaluated as of July 31, 1996, received full accreditation (Burns, Mandelker, and Northrup 1996).

Working with employer representatives, NCQA has developed the Health Plan Employer Data and Information Set (HEDIS) criteria, which purchasers and ultimately consumers can use in selecting health plans. The HEDIS criteria have undergone numerous modifications. To avoid development of multiple and possibly conflicting HEDIS criteria for commercial, Medicare, and Medicaid managed care enrollees, NCQA will develop a single HEDIS set that health plans can use for commercial and public managed care (Torta 1996).

Although critics of HEDIS have complained about its process orientation, in general, employers have been happy to have it. The 1996 HEDIS 3.0 version has 75 performance indicators, including new ones on health prevention and the quality of clinical care. It also focuses on major disease states such as cancer, heart disease, and diabetes. Health plans are now required to use a standard NCQA member satisfaction survey, not their own.

The Joint Commission has traditionally evaluated inpatient institutions. Because so many of those institutions have developed relationships with insurance partners and/or become part of integrated systems, the Joint Commission has expanded its scope to include health plans, PPOs, and integrated delivery systems. In 1997, the Joint Commission launched its new Oryx system, which will make performance measurement an integral part of evaluation efforts. By the end of the year, hospitals must select at least one approved system from the Joint Commission's approved list and identify and use at least two clinical measures that together address at least 20 percent of the patient population (Morrisey 1997).

Employer Strategies to Control Cost and Ensure Quality

In mature markets, employer strategies for cost control and quality assurance include but are not limited to restriction of insurance options; methodological evaluation of health insurance options; direct contracting; formation of purchasing coalitions; increase in employee cost sharing; creation of centers of excellence and carve-out products; sponsorship/support for demand management; and entry into the provision of care (Satinsky 1995a).

Restrictions in Choice of Health Insurance Options
Global competition has forced many U.S. companies to take a hard look at the absolute amount and percentage of dollars they spend on employee health care. To retain their own viability, many of them have reduced the number of health insurance offerings and given preference to managed care options that incorporate cost and utilization control into their structure and organization.

National employers that have taken this approach are Allied Signal and General Electric. In the automobile industry, Ford and Chrysler have supported a similar strategy; all new employees at these two companies must join an HMO to get employer-based coverage, according to a three-year contract signed by United Auto Workers (UAW) in 1996 (UAW 1996).

Not all employers, however, are willing to restrict employee choice of health insurance options. Some national employers and many small ones support multiple local options that offer high-quality care at low prices. For large employers, this approach can be administratively complex, but for midsize and small employers with relatively few locations, the administrative requirements of dealing with multiple plans can be manageable.

Methodological Evaluation of Health Insurance Options
The sophistication with which both public and private employers now evaluate health insurance options has changed dramatically. A decade ago, responsibility for the analysis of health insurance options and for making recommendations to management was probably buried within the human resources department. In small companies, the company treasurer or accountant might have done the job. Regardless of company size, health insurance generally received attention just once each year—when employers reviewed their offerings for the coming year.

Now health care costs receive top priority. In-house experts carefully evaluate options, monitor health care costs throughout the year, and work jointly with health plans, providers, and employees to control costs and ensure that quality meets mutually acceptable standards. Some employers hire an external specialist in network management such as UltraLink in California, Network Management Services in Minnesota, and Coventage in St. Louis (McCarthy 1996). These benefit management companies assist not only in the objective evaluation of options, but also with communications for new employees, health plan enrollment, eligibility reconciliation, reporting, member problems/complaints, and administration of flexible spending accounts, COBRA, and retirees.

In the public sector, one example of employer sophistication in managing health insurance is the California Public Employees Retirement System (CalPERS). CalPERS manages both the pension program and health plan for more than 900,000 lives, including employees, retirees, and dependents. Its scope of responsibility for health insurance includes contracting with HMOs, conducting health plan enrollment, paying premiums, arranging for a comprehensive set of services, and monitoring performance. In 1995, CalPERS employed 90 people working in enrollment and health plan administration (Hausner 1995).

In both private and public sectors, employer evaluation of health insurance options and performance has been aided by the development of state-of-the-art methods for measurement. By 1996, employers had access to three new methods for assessing quality and cost. CONQUEST 1.0 (Computerized Needs-Oriented Quality Measurement), developed by the Agency for Health Care Policy and Research (AHCPR), produces customized reports from two databases. The first contains information on clinical conditions and includes recommendations from AHCPR guidelines and other projects. The second database interlocks with the first and includes 1,200 clinical performance measures developed by multiple organizations (NCQA, the Joint Commission, and the Health Care Financing Administration [HCFA]). Employers also can purchase two proprietary methods, the Mercer Value Process and the Med-Score Value Purchasing Initiative. Both products can be tailored to measure the particular factors that an employer wants to monitor (New quality measures 1995).

Direct Contracting   Another employer approach to controlling health care costs and maintaining high-quality care is elimination of the health plan as the middle party. Historically, self-insured companies have been able to bypass insurance carriers and contract directly with providers. They used third-party administrators to handle administrative, marketing, and claims payment functions.

Direct contracting was encouraged by 1996 legislation regarding exclusive provider organizations (EPOs) and subsequent federal guidelines on provider-sponsored organizations (PSOs). Although skeptics contend that providers should not be in the health insurance business, many physicians, hospitals, and systems have perceived the new law as an opportunity to deal directly with purchasers and to assume internal responsibility for managing care.

Aside from legal issues, however, the wisdom of direct contracting is unclear. Some providers and systems lack the internal capacity and coordination to service multiple accounts. Others believe that direct contracting will jeopardize business that they receive through contractual arrangements with health plans. For example, by spring 1996, Friendly Hills HealthCare Network in La Habra, Calif., contracted with 20 health plans and believed that in its current market position, direct contracting could negatively affect the number of covered lives for which it was responsible (Friendly Hills 1996).

Formation of Purchasing Coalitions   Purchasers at national, regional, and local levels have joined together to analyze health care costs, maintain data, and negotiate with providers. Although the health insurance purchasing coalition concept predates President Clinton's advocacy of the idea in his 1993 health reform proposals, the potential of national health reform certainly encouraged the formation of coalitions in many communities.

Two important national developments occurred in 1995. A small group of major employers banded together to form the National HMO Purchasing Coalition. The new group included American Express, Merrill Lynch, Pfizer, Inc., Marriott International, Nabisco Brands Inc., IBM, ITT, Sears, and two other companies that preferred anonymity (Presenting 1995). The coalition represented 600,000 covered lives and was expected to purchase $1 billion of health care services throughout the country. Within a year after its formation, the coalition released information on the methodology used to select health plans: 30 percent of the equation was related to cost and 70 percent was related to quality (How the big guys rank HMOs 1996).

In the other national development, the Foundation for Accountability, known as FACCT, was formed by leading purchasers.

(Winslow 1995). The new group represented major public and private purchasers, including HCFA. It identified five major diseases for which it would define quality of care delivered by HMOs: asthma, coronary artery disease, breast cancer, diabetes, and low back pain. To achieve its goal, FACCT developed a process to review current medical literature, identify quality indicators, endorse quality measurement sets, and encourage use by purchasers and consumers (Burns, Mandelker, and Northrup 1996).

Regional coalition activity has been strong. In Minneapolis–St. Paul, following an unsuccessful attempt to influence the passage of favorable legislation, influential employers formed the Buyers Healthcare Action Group (BHCAG) in 1992. By 1996, BHCAG included 23 employers, including such giants as General Motors, Pillsbury, 3M, and the state of Minnesota.

BHCAG's strategy has evolved. At first, members developed a common self-insured health plan and a POS option. The group then contracted with a small number of systems and with 50 medical groups. Employers and providers jointly supported the creation of the Institute for Clinical Systems Integration to encourage health plans to demonstrate commitment to cost and quality management. BHCAG was able to reduce health care costs and to increase employee satisfaction with both medical services and health plan administration (Kemnitz 1996). Yet BHCAG was not satisfied with the level of competition. Beginning in January 1997, the group expected to implement another innovative approach in which teams of caregivers would compete for consumers based on price and quality of care provided (Health care 1996). BHCAG hopes that its new strategy will foster more competition than dealing with large managed care plans, most of which had overlapping provider participation.

The Greater Cleveland Health Quality Choice Coalition, a buyer coalition that predates President Clinton's talk of health insurance purchasing cooperatives, is a well-known regional purchasing coalition. In 1994, the coalition released its fourth report on hospital performance and expected that the data would enable assessment of the quality and value of care provided by 29 participating institutions (Employers 1995).

Employers organized into purchasing coalitions have influenced not only provider performance but also health plan performance and pricing. For example, in San Francisco, an 11-member coalition that was part of the larger Bay Area Business Group on Health obtained rate concessions from more than a dozen HMOs

(Kenkel 1994). It also linked premium payment to health plan ability to meet criteria for customer service, quality of care, and data reporting. Other coalitions that have directly influenced health plans are the Central Florida Health Care Coalition, the Memphis Business Group on Health, and the Colorado Health Purchasing Alliance (Hausner 1995).

Employee Cost Sharing   Employers that have asked employees to share costs for health insurance have anticipated an impact on behavior. Companies that were once reluctant to pass on cost sharing to employees and dependents have moved away from their role as "benevolent provider." Many now require employees to make co-payments for office visits, emergency room visits, and prescription drugs. More positive approaches to employee cost sharing have included financial incentives for participation in exercise and health education programs.

Creation of Centers of Excellence and Carve-Outs   A number of employers, particularly national ones with locations in multiple sites, have adopted a centers-of-excellence approach to control costs and ensure quality in high-cost complex cases. Carve-out benefits resemble the center-of-excellence approach in that the benefit is separated out from the mainstream method for delivery of care. The distinction is that carve-outs are not only delivered differently but also are usually insured separately.

Although it can be argued that both approaches perpetuate the existing fragmentation of health care financing and delivery, both the centers-of-excellence and carve-out strategies have remained viable and have often saved dollars spent on care. Common applications are organ transplantation, advanced cardiac care, and mental health and substance abuse.

Delta Airlines, for example, used a competitive bidding process to select six cardiac programs throughout the country to provide care for 72,000 employees (Leavenworth 1994). With regard to mental health and substance abuse, many employers and health plans believe that these two problems are unusually costly and difficult to manage. Rather than include them within their basic health insurance plan, employers treat them as a separate benefit that is managed and often insured by a specialized company.

Sponsorship/Support for Demand Management
Demand management has a variety of meanings. Generically, the

term often applies to the development of methods for responding to marketplace demands (such as questions, concerns, and complaints) from health plan enrollees, referring clinicians, and/or the general public. Many employers have sponsored or supported demand management programs that respond to employees' questions and that facilitate appropriate use of the health care system.

As an example, one employer looked carefully at employees who repeatedly sought emergency room care for symptoms that could more appropriately be treated in other settings. Common causes, particularly for young parents, were fear, inexperience with parenting, and reluctance to wait for an office appointment. The employer, the health plan that insured most of its employees, and several providers jointly sponsored a toll-free telephone line that employees could access on a 24-hour basis. Over time, employees learned to use the new telephone resource to obtain information or assistance in accessing the appropriate level of care. Consequently, the number of inappropriate visits to the emergency room decreased.

Employer Development of Health Care Services   Some employers have given up on the health care delivery system and decided to produce rather than purchase health care services (Solovy 1994). Delta Airlines, for example, has built a primary care center near Hartsfield International Airport in Atlanta. The John Deere Family Healthplan in Des Moines, Iowa, has developed primary care centers that provide services to both company employees and to employees of other companies. Although these programs have met employer clinical and financial goals, they are exceptions, not the rule. Most employers have left delivery and coordination of health care services to providers.

REIMBURSEMENT

Reimbursement (the method by which payers pay for health care) is another external factor that has stimulated the growth of integrated systems. Payers competing in global markets watched health care costs and the rate of cost increase grow beyond their ability to pay. Both private and public sector payers were unwilling to shoulder the entire burden of paying for as much care as providers delivered. They limited the growth of health care costs and shifted financial risk.

In mature managed care markets, health plans, insurers, and providers agree to accept financial risk for the care they provide to specific populations. The three common methods by which providers are paid under risk arrangements are capitation payment, percentage of premium, and the use of incentives and bonuses designed to reward efficient delivery of care and quality outcomes.

Capitation

Capitation is a method of paying for care based on the following five assumptions:

- Enrollees who sign up with a health plan, health system, or any other entity that accepts financial risk for their care belong to that entity.
- Based on demographic characteristics such as age and sex, it is possible to budget in advance the cost per member per month that the capitated entity will incur to care for its members.
- The expected monthly cost of enrollees is a finite amount; if the actual cost of care exceeds the budget, there is no recourse for additional funding.
- Protections can be built into capitation payments so that care for individuals or for episodes of illness that exceed a particular dollar amount are covered by reinsurance rather than by the capitation payment.
- Success under capitation requires management of health and wellness in addition to illness.

Providers who agree to accept capitation payment have choices in the financial arrangements. To make sure they have a large enough enrollment base over which to spread financial risk, they can establish a minimum number of enrollees for which they accept capitation. They also have options in the scope of capitation. Sometimes primary care providers are capitated, but specialists and facilities are reimbursed under different reimbursement methods. In other cases, specialists but not primary care providers are capitated. Or, all providers and facilities are capitated. There can be variations in the distribution of capitated dollars for different services. In general, when primary care physicians are capitated, they receive a sufficient proportion of the total capitation to cover their responsibilities for providing and coordinating care. Some payers recognize the management or "gatekeeper" responsibility of primary care providers by paying a monthly management fee in addition to the capitated payment.

Percentage of Premium

Percentage of premium also allows payers to shift financial risk to providers. Some providers prefer it to capitation because they have more flexibility in determining the distribution of dollars. Under this arrangement, payers and payees agree in advance that a particular percentage of the health care premium will be turned over to providers. The providers then determine the division of the dollar, the management of care, and the distribution of surplus/deficits that occur.

Incentives and Bonuses

Financial incentives and bonuses are yet another way to encourage providers to behave in a certain way as they deliver and coordinate care. For example, given the symbiotic relationship between physicians and other sites of care, physicians can be rewarded for reducing acute care utilization and for increasing other types of care. Or, physicians and other caregivers can be rewarded based on service standards, clinical outcomes, and enrollee satisfaction.

In less developed managed care markets, providers do not assume financial risk. Compensation for care remains completely or partially tied to the units of care produced or delivered (for example, visits, tests, consultations). There are no fixed monthly payments; instead providers are paid on a fee-for-service basis or some variation that rewards them for the volume of patients whom they treat.

Most of the country is neither fully capitated nor fully fee-for-service, but functions somewhere in between the two extremes. Existing evidence suggests that this "middle-of-the-road" status creates great confusion for providers. If they receive capitation for some but not all of their enrollees/patients, do they provide care differently for the different groups? Many providers claim that when they are at financial risk for 35 percent or more of their patients, they begin to practice as if all people are under risk arrangements.

Although providers throughout the country have responded to increasing external pressure to accept financial risk, without national health reform, it is unlikely that everyone will be fully capitated. Even in states that already have high penetrations of managed care in both private and public sectors, there is variation. For example, by 1996, California was one of the most tightly managed care states in the country, with capitation as the dominant form of payment. But Massachusetts, another state with a high penetration of managed care, is not moving in the direction of full capitation. Health plans believe that provider costs are still too high and that they can continue to exert pressure. Only when payers believe they can no longer reduce the cost of care are they likely to move toward capitation.

EXPECTATIONS FOR DELIVERY AND COORDINATION OF CARE

In mature managed care environments, the delivery and coordination of health care services are responsive to the external expectations of the marketplace, not to the internal preferences of providers themselves.

The important expectations that the external market now places on the delivery system include provision/coordination of a continuum of care, emphasis on alternatives to inpatient hospitalization, coordination/collaboration of administrative and clinical aspects of care, and demonstration of quality and outcomes.

The continuum of care concept includes health care services that are delivered at different points in time and in different locations. Enrollees may move from one part of the continuum to another, but they never really leave it. The market expects the delivery system to pay close attention to health and wellness as well as to the treatment of illness.

The notion of a continuum of care implies options. Not all care must be delivered in an inpatient hospital setting. The market expects the delivery system to develop alternatives for care and make every possible effort to steer enrollees to the appropriate setting. Hospitals that are instrumental in the formation of integrated delivery systems often have difficulty accepting this reality.

If integrated systems are just old relationships with new names, market expectations will be disappointed. Integration implies coordination and collaboration of administrative and clinical aspects of care. For example, can system enrollees contact a single point in the system where they are triaged to the appropriate point of care? Do system case managers work with enrollees regardless of where they access care? Although a system claims to offer a continuum of care, must enrollees register and reregister every time they access different system components? Are the clinical results of care rendered in one part of the system shared with others? Faced with these difficult questions, many providers have chosen to integrate vertically.

Finally, regarding quality and outcomes, can integrated systems respond to payer-generated standards, or do they focus only on internally generated measurements? How willing are they to collaboratively set new parameters?

External pressures on the health care delivery system are indeed great. The creation of integrated health care systems has the potential to meet these expectations, but that is only a starting point. Their legal existence does not guarantee that they will meet their goals or external expectations.

References

The Advisory Board Company. 1994. *Quality measures: Next generation of outcomes tracking.* Vol. 2. Washington, D.C.: The Advisory Board Company.

Allina may cover alternative therapies to meet consumer demand in twin cities. 1996. *BNAs Managed Care Reporter* 2 (46): 1113–1114 (20 November).

Banks, P. G. 1995. Physician practice acquisition. Presentation at Centralized Practice Plan Directors Round Table, 11 September.

Boston system bucks the trend and woos capitation. 1996. *Hospital Managed Care Strategies* 4 (5): 53–55 (May).

Burns, J., J. Mandelker, and L. Northrup. 1996. Buyers shift their focus to quality improvement. *Managed Healthcare* 6 (12): 24–27 (December).

Carriers rely on managed care to slash work comp costs. 1996. *Workers Comp Report* 2 (3): 1.

Cochrane, J. 1996. The California consolidation game. *Integrated Healthcare Report* 1–8 (July).

Employers go to bed with Cleveland's latest performance report. 1995. *Report on medical guidelines and outcomes research* 6 (1): 5–7 (12 January).

Friendly Hills HealthCare Network. 1996. Duke University Medical Center site visit, 6 May.

Harvard Pilgrim to acquire Matthew Thornton for $75 million. 1997. *BNAs Managed Care Reporter* 3 (2): 39 (8 January).

Hausner, T. 1995. Purchasing coalitions and managed care. *Managed Care Quarterly* 3 (1): 76–88 (winter).

Health care market's third stage will increase competition, quality. 1996. *BNAs Managed Care Reporter* 2 (42): 1012 (23 October).

How the big guys rank HMOs. 1996. *Business and Health* 14 (11): 16 (November).

Integrated disability slices costs in half. 1996. *Business and Health* 14 (11): 12 (November).

Kemnitz, D. 1996. What employers are looking for. Presentation at 32nd Annual National Forum on Hospital and Health Affairs, 15 May, at Duke University, Durham, N.C.

Kenkel, P. 1994. *Straight As: How to use quality report cards to win market share.* New York: Thompson Publishing Group.

Leavenworth, G. 1994. Four cost-cutting strategies. *Business and Health* 12 (8): 26–34 (August).

McCarthy, R. 1996. Who should be managing your managed care plans? *Business and Health* 14 (5): 25–29 (May).

Merging toward market domination. 1996. *Business and Health* 14 (5): 16 (May).

Morrissey, J. 1995. Opposition stalls N.H. HMO merger. *Modern Healthcare* 25 (27): 38 (25 September).

———. 1997. Quality measures hit prime time. *Modern Health-care* 27 (18): 66–76 (5 May).

New quality measures abound. 1995. *Business and Health* 13 (5):12–17 (May).

Oxford goes new age. 1996. *Business and Health* 14 (11): 13 (November).

Pham, A. 1996. HMO will combine products. *Boston Globe,* 5 April, 57, 67.

Presenting the first nationwide health coalition. 1995. *Business and Health* 13 (6): 13 (June).

Satinsky, M. A. 1995a. Advanced practice nurse in a managed care environment. In *Advanced practice nursing,* by J. V. Hickey, R. M. Ouimette, and S. L. Venegeni. Philadelphia: Lippincott.

———. 1995b. *An executive guide to case management strategies.* Chicago: American Hospital Publishing, Inc.

Shortell, S.M., R. R. Gillies, D. A. Anderson, K. M. Erickson, and J. B. Mitchell. 1996. *Remaking healthcare in America: Build-ing organized delivery systems.* San Francisco: Jossey-Bass Publishers.

Solovy, A. 1994. New power strategies (the battle for control). *Hospitals and Health Networks* 68 (24): 24–34.

Torta, P. 1996. Quality initiatives: Medicaid HEDIS and ensuring access for Medicaid. Presentation at National Managed Care Congress, Washington, D.C., 30 April.

UAW drives new hires into HMOs. 1996. *Business and Health* 14 (11): 10 (November).

Winslow, R. 1995. Care at HMOs to be rated by new system. *Wall Street Journal,* 25 September, B14.

CHAPTER

3

Developing Integrated Health Care

INTRODUCTION

Health care professionals searching for a cookbook on integrated health care systems have a dilemma. Although large conglomerates in industry are relatively common, systems are relatively new in health care. The majority of organizations that call themselves integrated health care systems did not start that way, and their evolution is incomplete. Much of the early research on integration in health care has relied on case studies. For example, researchers at Northwestern University, Chicago, and BBC Research & Consulting in Denver have collectively looked at 21 systems (figs. 3-1 and 3-2). Findings from both efforts were published in 1996 (Shortell and others 1996; Coddington and others 1996). Also, a ranking of the top 100 systems (fig. 3-3) has been published by St. Anthony Publishing Company; also, Ernst & Young has released the results of a survey of more than 200 systems (St. Anthony Publishing Company 1996; Ernst & Young 1996). Northwestern University and the Hospital Research and Educational Trust are planning a more formalized project on the structural and strategic elements of newly emerging health care organizations that have been organized around hospitals.

Although there is much to be learned from existing systems as well as those that have stumbled and fallen along the way, it is

FIGURE 3-1.   Integrated Systems Included in 1996
Northwestern University Study

Baylor Health Care System (Dallas, Tex.)
EHS Health Care (Oak Brook, Ill.—presently Advocate Health
   Care, resulting from a merger of EHS and Lutheran General
   Health System in January 1995)
Fairview Hospital and Healthcare Services (Minneapolis–St.
   Paul, Minn.)
Franciscan Health System (Aston, Penn.)
Henry Ford Health System (Detroit, Mich.)
Mercy Health Services (Farmington Hills, Mich.)
Sentara Health System (Norfolk, Va.)
Sharp HealthCare (San Diego, Calif.)
Sisters of Providence Health System (Seattle, Wash.)
Sutter Health (Sacramento, Calif.)
UniHealth (Burbank, Calif.)

Source: Shortell, S. M., R. R. Gillies, A. A. Anderson, K. M. Erickson, and
J. B. Mitchell. 1996. *Remaking health care in America: Building organized delivery
systems.* San Francisco: Jossey-Bass, Inc.

important to evaluate their experiences within a broader context.
The development and growth of integrated health care systems is
a *process*, not an act or a series of activities. A major challenge for
most systems is to envision that process and treat it as the context
into which many activities must fit and link together.

   This chapter describes the generic process of creating, maintaining, and continually fine-tuning integrated health care systems—that
is, the journey of integration. As they evolve, systems address three
macro issues: market forces, organization, and internal functions.
They repeatedly address each one, *revisiting* them at different points
in time. Simultaneously, systems progress from one growth stage to
another, building sequentially and moving on to subsequent challenges (Jones and Mayerhofer 1994). Figure 3-4 shows the macro
issues, the growth stages, and the relationships between the two.

MACRO ISSUES

Throughout their evolution, systems repeatedly focus on market
forces, organizational structure, and internal focus. As systems

FIGURE 3-2.   Integrated Systems Included in 1996 BBC
Research & Consulting Study*

Advocate Health Care (Park Ridge, Ill.)
Aetna Professional Management Corporation (Glastonbury,
    Conn.)
Baptist Health System (Birmingham, Ala.)
Bassett Health Systems (Cooperstown, N.Y.)
Columbia/HCA (Nashville, Tenn.)
Columbia/HCA
HealthSystem Minnesota (Minneapolis, Minn.)
Intermountain Health Care (Salt Lake City, Utah)
Lovelace Health Systems (Albuquerque, N.M.)
The Nalle Clinic (Charlotte, N.C.)
Scott & White (Temple, Tex.)

*Published by Center for Research in Ambulatory Health Care Administration,
Englewood, Colo.

Source: Coddington, D. C., C. R. Chapman, and K. M. Pokowski. 1996. *Making
integrated health care work.* Englewood, Colo.: Center for Ambulatory Health Care
Administration.

FIGURE 3-3.   Top 10 Integrated Delivery Systems as Ranked
by St. Anthony Publishing, Inc.

Rank	System
1	Daughters of Charity National Health System
2	Kaiser Permanente (Southern California Region)
3	Catholic Healthcare West
4	Kaiser Permanente (Northern California Region)
5	Henry Ford Health System
6	Allina Health System
7	Advocate Health Care
8	Intermountain Health Care
9	Mercy Health Services
10	Catholic Health Care Network

Note: The proprietary ranking system is based on business, not quality, factors.

Source: *Integrated healthcare 100 directory.* 1996. Reston, Va.: St. Anthony
Publishing.

FIGURE 3-4. Evolution of Regional Health Care Systems

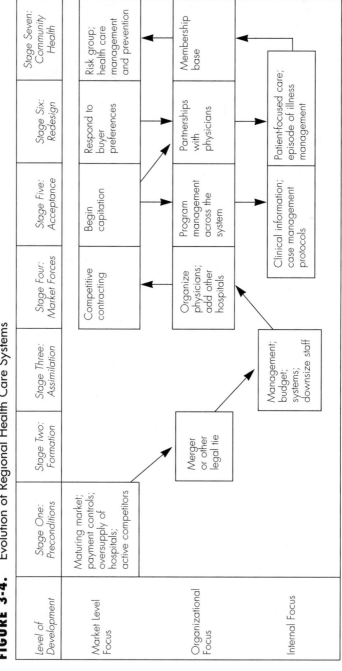

Source: Jones, W. J., and J. J. Mayerhofer. 1994. Regional health care systems: Implications for health care reform. *Managed Care Quarterly* 2(1): 31–44.

move through subsequent stages of growth, those three issues interact with, conflict with, and influence one another.

Market Forces

As explained in chapter 2, the external market plays an important role in systems development. In less mature managed care markets, providers feel minimal pressure from employers, insurers, and consumers. They continue to provide health care in traditional ways. As markets move toward maturity, providers and insurers, alone or collaboratively, respond to pressures to manage the cost and quality of care. They are encouraged to integrate service delivery, accept financial risk, and pay more attention to the needs and demands of payers and consumers.

Market forces impact integrated systems throughout their evolution. At the outset, they can be strong stimuli for systems formation. At later stages, the market reacts to what systems have put in place. Market satisfaction/dissatisfaction and market competition then influence systems thinking. In more mature managed care markets, the external market again generates certain expectations that systems must meet. (See case 6-4 for examples.)

Organizational Structure

All integrated health care systems grapple with the challenge of creating an organization. Because organization may be the first activity in which previously unrelated parties participate, it offers the potential for both positive opportunity and peril. Preoccupation with "sizing each other up," internal politics, and the designation of senior leadership may consume so much energy that participants neglect the important issues that must be addressed after the system is legally in place. The complexities of bringing multiple organizations together and the embryonic state of industry knowledge contribute to the difficulty of systems organization.

Important considerations in organizing any integrated system include the following:

- System goals
- Legal and regulatory issues

- Provider network issues: which providers? how many providers? what mix of providers?
- Ownership versus contractual relationships (that is, virtual integration or actual ownership)
- For-profit or not-for-profit status
- Capital requirements
- Insurance partner issues

System Goals   Ideally, integrated health care delivery systems, with or without the financing component, achieve consensus on long- and short-term goals *before* making other decisions that may facilitate or obstruct their achievement. They revisit those goals periodically and monitor the progress and appropriateness of system direction. If necessary, goals are modified. System structures and operations change to accommodate original and modified goals.

In reality, however, many integrated health care systems do not set goals first. According to the 1996 Ernst & Young survey of integrated delivery and financing systems, 10 percent of the respondents had no strategic plan, and 61 percent had a plan that covered only three years (Ernst & Young 1996). Unfortunately many developing systems have assumed that the ultimate goal is to create a health care system. They do not understand that an integrated system, with or without a financing component, is a means to an end, rather than an end in and of itself. Presumably that end will bear some relationship to the improvement of the health and wellness of populations and individuals (see chapter 4).

System sponsorship has a major impact on system goals. If a system is hospital- or physician-initiated and/or dominated, its goals are likely to reflect the priorities of the provider community. If a system is sponsored and/or dominated by a health plan or insurance company, system goals will be different. Hybrid systems that integrate both health care delivery and financing have goals that reflect a combination of provider and insurer interests.

For example, hospital-sponsored systems frequently identify expansion of the continuum of care as a major goal. Although many acute care hospitals have already diversified their services, others lack the resources and/or relationships needed to offer the entire continuum of care (Japsen 1996). Involvement in a system may facilitate and accelerate development of the missing pieces.

Another common goal in hospital-driven systems is the involvement of physicians in leadership roles. Although there is general recognition of the importance of strong physician-hospital relationships, the opportunity to participate in systems development may provide a context in which physicians can emerge as strong leaders at the governance, administrative, and operational levels.

Providers that are experiencing shrinking revenues and increasing costs may view systems as a way to reverse that trend. Thus, another goal for provider-driven systems may be to increase revenues and reduce costs.

Access to capital is another common goal for development of an integrated health care system. For example, small providers, single-service providers (such as rehabilitation and long-term care), and providers in rural areas may experience financial difficulties and seek collaborative efforts as a potential source of capital. Likewise, some of the mega-mergers in California in 1996 were designed to improve access to capital.

Academic medical centers/systems (AMCs) that are involved in the formation of integrated health care delivery and/or financing systems generally become involved for all the reasons that other providers do—with two additions. First, most AMCs are dependent on public sector patients (Medicaid and Medicare) to sustain their teaching programs. Rather than risk the loss of this important patient base, they may focus on improving the overall health of these groups of patients. Second, the historical balance between teaching, research, and patient care becomes precarious in highly competitive markets, and AMCs need to create ways to address losses in clinical revenue that previously supported teaching and research. Participation in health care systems may enable them to build and formalize networks, turn their attention to population-based care, and apply research findings to improvements in clinical care.

Payer-initiated systems often identify such goals as economies of scale, reduction of duplication of services, more efficient contracting, and alignment of physician and hospital incentives. Those payers that were in the managed care (not the indemnity) business generally have less difficulty setting system goals. By contrast, indemnity companies must understand risk and responsibility for population-based care in order to function as systems.

Finally, integrated systems that combine both the delivery and financing of health care generally incorporate all the previously described goals.

Legal and Regulatory Issues   All systems must address
legal and regulatory issues, including but not limited to antitrust

fraud and abuse, taxation, and laws applying to licensure and the corporate practice of medicine. As suggested in chapter 5 and described in the appendix, astute anticipation of these issues can minimize delays in the process of integration and avoid creation of barriers. In addition to the appendix, another good resource on legal issues for integrated systems is Randall's 1996 executive guide (Randall 1996).

Provider Network Issues   At least three provider network issues receive attention when systems organize: (1) Which providers participate? (2) How many providers are necessary to care for the target population? (3) What mix of providers best suits both supply and demand? All three issues are affected by a critical but unknown factor—the impact of medical technology on treatment and communications among different sites of care.

Which providers? Ideally, when integrated health care systems form, they match their system capacity to population needs. In reality, decisions about which providers participate are usually a combination of reason and politics. Important factors are geography, prior existence of "pre-systems" structures, capital, and provider performance.

The impact of geography on provider participation in integrated systems has received less emphasis than it deserves. Advances in telecommunications have convinced many systems to "go big." The ease and speed with which information can cross natural geographic boundaries and state lines can blur the importance of health care as a local business. Wiser systems, however, understand that national presence is not inconsistent with regionalized management that is more responsive to local health needs and to the concerns of individual patients.

The existence of pre-systems structures also impacts systems' decisions as to which providers participate in a network. For example, PHOs frequently emerge as a first step toward the development of larger regional systems. Sometimes these PHOs link with one another and create a "super PHO," which might then become the foundation of a large regional system.

Availability and sources of capital both influence the selection of providers in integrated systems, particularly in the early stages of development. Fledgling systems generally lack the operating experience needed to raise outside capital. If they seek financial backing within the provider community, the power of the purse may impact which providers participate in the system.

Finally, as integrated systems mature, information on provider performance may enable them to be more selective about provider participation. Especially when systems are at financial risk, they may decide that care should be delivered by fewer people or organizations. An example is the Brigham and Women's PHO in Boston. That academic medical center has historically not limited specialist referrals to a subset of its physicians. For risk-contracting arrangements, however, not all specialists receive referrals.

How many providers? System decisions regarding the number of providers can, but do not always, relate to the size, location, and demographic characteristics of the population for which that system expects to assume responsibility. Ideally, a system should provide an accessible continuum of care for a specific population in a prescribed geographic area; the number of providers should relate to need. However, like decisions relating to provider participation, if a system is provider initiated and the provider community is the source of capital, initial overcapacity may be tolerated.

Even when systems are methodical about "right-sizing" themselves, defining accessibility of care is a subjective exercise. For example, because of an undersupply of primary care physicians, people in underserved rural areas may be accustomed to driving long distances for care. A system serving this population might weigh two options. It might expand the provider network by encouraging use of midlevel practitioners, or it might maintain the status quo because of residents' customary health-seeking behavior.

What professional mix of providers? Integrated systems use both external standards and subjective judgment to determine the desirable mix of providers. With respect to the "right" ratio of primary care to specialist physicians, a common target in a mature managed care environment is a 50:50 ratio. In an aggressive integrated system, that ratio may be as high as 64:46. Systems that start from a primary care base may be sized properly from the outset. Likewise, systems that are initiated by a health plan rather than by providers may be appropriately sized. Provider-initiated systems such as Lovelace Health Systems in New Mexico, Duke University Medical Center & Health System in North Carolina, and Partners HealthCare System in Massachusetts may need to resize themselves over time. Case 6-5 provides a brief snapshot of the way in which these three systems have addressed primary care capacity.

In most systems, factors other than target ratios impact decisions about the professional mix of providers. For example, if systems identify managing the total health of a population as a goal, they have choices about the types of providers they engage. If they have highly developed case or care management components, they may rely on these professionals for disease prevention, wellness, and health promotion. At St. Mary's Hospital and Health Center in Tucson, for example, nurse case managers provide and coordinate care in an ambulatory setting of community health centers. There is close collaboration between the case managers and the client population and strong emphasis on enrollee responsibility for maintaining health and wellness. At Friendly Hills HealthCare Network, the case management system includes primary care, clinical nurse specialist, hospital, and geriatric case managers. At each point where case managers and enrollees come into contact, there is emphasis on disease prevention, health promotion, and enrollee awareness of health and wellness (Satinsky 1995).

Other integrated systems, however, take different approaches to disease prevention, wellness, and health promotion. In systems that include both health care delivery and financing, health plan staff may assume responsibility for those activities, often but not always in conjunction with provider staff who also perform these functions.

Systems have different philosophies about the types of providers who should provide care. In some systems that have an adequate supply of primary care physicians, only physicians provide primary care. Other systems make good use of midlevel practitioners such as nurse practitioners and physician assistants.

Ownership versus Contractual Relationships One of the major points of contention in the development of integrated health care systems is the ownership versus contractual relationship (that is, virtual integration) issue, described in chapter 1. Arguments can be made for both approaches, and there are many examples of each. The proponents of each point of view are adamant about their opinions; they agree only on the conclusion that it is too soon to know which approach will have the better result.

Advocates of ownership contend that as integrated systems grow, the only effective way for components to relate to one another is through common ownership. They contend that without the linkage of common ownership, it is difficult if not impossible to align financial incentives, develop effective management information systems, respond to concerns of consumers and payers, and accept a single check from a public or private payer. In my experience, mergers, acquisitions, joint ventures and all that go with them do not, by definition, address the people part. These legal acts are only a starting point. They may make some decisions easier than others, but they do not eliminate the need to attentively cultivate relationships at all levels.

Kaiser Permanente built its reputation on ownership—prior to 1990. A consistent strategy for employing physicians and owning facilities enabled Kaiser to grow and thrive when other plans suffered during the 1986–87 health insurance crash. By the early 1990s, however, the ownership strategy no longer worked. Facing losses in market share in its major Pacific markets and elsewhere, Kaiser adopted a more flexible approach and included in its delivery system networks physicians who practice in their private offices. In 1996, physicians in 12 separate Permanente Medical Groups formed a national federation, PermCorp. Among the new organization's goals was to provide management of services to non-Kaiser physicians. Kaiser took another nontraditional step toward virtual integration by eliminating inpatient services at some of its hospitals and contracting with community hospitals. In yet another departure from Kaiser's historical pattern of ownership, Kaiser Permanente Northwest Division and Group Health Cooperative of Puget Sound entered into merger discussions.

The virtual integration advocates are equally adamant about their position—that *relationships,* not ownership, create effective integration. Proponents of this approach cite the negative experience of private industry and contend that asset mergers and acquisitions do not guarantee success. They contend that integration involves relationships among *people,* within and outside integrated systems.

Friendly Hills HealthCare Network and Humana are examples of virtual integration. Friendly Hills admits patients to 12 hospitals but owns only one of them. Physicians in the Friendly Hills Medical Group and in the staff model practices acquired from CIGNA have been integrated into a single new group. Other physicians organized into IPAs have contractual relationships. Humana made a major decision in 1992 when it sold its hospitals to Columbia/HCA. Today Humana and Columbia/HCA have contractual marketing relationships.

In their early stages of growth, some systems prefer a mixed and flexible approach; they own some but not all of the components. For example, between 1992 and 1996, Duke developed important virtual relationships with a major insurer and with several major suppliers. Financial incentives were aligned. Simultaneously with its emphasis on relationship building, Duke purchased some components of its system. For example, enhancement of primary care capacity involved the acquisition of primary care physicians.

The mixed strategy can be very effective in the early stages of system growth. It allows a system to experiment gradually with different approaches. If early ownership experiences are positive for both parties, the system can use them as a model for developing other similar linkages. On the other hand, if ownership results in mutual dissatisfaction, the system can examine its problems before moving ahead. The gradual approach to ownership and relationship building can help systems understand what it means to collaborate with other organizations.

For-Profit or Not-for-Profit Status An important issue that developing systems must address is whether or not to operate as for-profit, not-for-profit, or hybrid organizations. Access to capital and tax status are the obvious but not the only differences. Proponents of the for-profit approach highlight the ability of proprietary organizations to make quick decisions, consolidate operations, downsize work forces, increase outpatient services, and respond quickly to payer demands for steep price concessions (Greene and Lutz 1996). Advocates of the not-for-profit approach cite the potential negative impact of for-profit systems: dumping uninsured patients, taking dollars out of local communities, avoiding subsidization of education and research, amassing huge personal fortunes, and creating conflict of interest situations that pit patient care and stockholder profit against each other (Friedman 1996).

Somewhere between the not-for-profit and for-profit extremes are integrated systems that incorporate elements of both types of entities. These hybrid organizations may "offer the strength, speed, and capital of proprietaries, along with the strong values, stability, and community orientation of the mission-driven organization" (Flower 1996). When the partners have the right chemistry, the hybrids have a healthy tension that can be very successful. Examples of hybrid organizations are Tulane University Medical Center in New Orleans and Methodist in San Antonio, Tex. These systems are described in case 6-6.

Capital Requirements Throughout their evolution, integrated health care delivery/financing systems must deal with the issue of capital. Following are the most commonly asked questions:

- How much money is needed?
- From what source(s) will financing come?

In general, the amount of capital that is needed is directly related to system sponsorship/structure and phase in system development. For example, if a system includes both a health care delivery system and a health plan, by the time the two come together as a system, the health plan may already have made major financial investments in activities such as claims processing, quality assurance, and marketing. Although costly changes may be needed, initial investment already has occurred.

However, if a system is initiated and sponsored by a health care delivery system, investments in activities that are traditionally insurance functions are less likely to have been made. In most but not all provider-initiated systems, early capital investments are likely to be directed toward development of a health care delivery system, not infrastructure. Graduate Health System in Philadelphia, a hospital-initiated system that made an unusually early commitment to information systems, was an exception (GHS links 1995).

Not all systems that are initiated by delivery systems have similar capital needs; some are further along than others. For example, systems that evolve from early-stage integration organizations such as MSOs or PHOs have greater needs than systems that evolve from more advanced-stage multispecialty group practices.

A system's stage of development has a direct impact on its capital needs and sources of capital. For example, a pre-operational system needs funding to build a system. It needs to pay for market surveys and market research, consultation, legal fees, and actuarial assistance. At this early point in its development, the emerging system may have little or no revenue, no securing assets, and minimal opportunity to raise capital short of participant investment. At the other end of the evolutionary spectrum, a mature system with a strong record of profitability and debt repayment can more easily acquire new capital to support its needs (fig. 3-5).

The implication of these differences is great. In markets where newer systems compete with more mature ones, there are likely to be real differences in system priorities and outcomes. Purchasers (that is, employers and/or consumers) with clear expectations of cost, quality, and service may have very distinct options.

In addition to questions about the amount and sources of capital, two other important issues must be addressed. One is the relationship of system goals to capital, and the other is an integrated system's use of capital (fig. 3-6).

FIGURE 3-5.   Suggested Focuses of Capital Planning
at Different Stages of Systems Development

Early
    Organization/Development
    Consultation
    Legal
    Accounting
    Delivery System Development/Management
        Practice Acquisition: Primary Care and/or Specialists
    Operating Cash
    Early Information Systems (IS) Development

Midphase
    Maintain System as Viable Business

Mature
    Enhance/expand core business
    Add critical related business

At many different times—start-up, midphase, and mature
phase—systems develop goals and determine the financial feasibility of their plans. Not all systems designs and strategies are financially feasible, however, and financial reality may force a system to
modify or scale down its original plans. Often systems may believe
that a merger will mutually improve access to capital. Some not-for-
profit systems link with for-profit organizations for the same reason.
Although such shifts in system strategies may facilitate access to
desirable financial resources, they may also dramatically change the
focus and course of the new organization.

Another important issue related to capitalization of integrated
systems is the use of the money. The health care industry is accustomed to spending resources on tangible assets; large percentages
of the health care dollar have been spent on facilities, supplies, and
equipment. As a result, when providers sponsor integrated systems,
they may expect that they will use capital in systems development
in a similar way. They may overlook an important point that the
health insurance industry understands better—that is, that intangi-
ble assets such as relationships, contracts, and trade names may be
more relevant in creating value for consumers and employers.

FIGURE 3-6.   Options for Capitalizing Health Care Integrated Delivery Systems

Use Own Money	Use Someone Else's Money
Physicians Hospitals Local Employers	Equity —Venture capital —Initial public offering —Public company stock
	Debt —Bond market —Bank —Other lenders

Source: Medimetrix Group, 1996

Expertise in organizational development, ongoing staff training, and cultural change are all essential to the successful development of integrated health care systems. However, those intangibles do not always receive attention and financial support.

Insurance Partner Issues   One of the important questions that developing systems must answer is whether or not to include both delivery system and financing components. Systems take different approaches. Some are philosophically opposed to linking health care delivery and financing; they steer clear of such arrangements. Other systems link delivery and financing as a short-term strategy to gain control of market share. They then sell off all or a portion of the health plan component to a larger plan, reaping a financial benefit. By then, enrollee loyalty has already developed. Still other systems bounce back and forth, alternating between the linkage and separation of health care delivery and financing (Kertesz 1996). Figures 3-7 and 3-8 list integrated health care systems that have approached the separation or combination of the delivery and financing of care in different ways; refer to case 6-7 for examples.

Many systems do not address the insurance issue directly. They suffer from "organizational schizophrenia" because they are unclear as to whether they are in the provider and/or the insurance business (Mead-Fox and Scheur 1996). As a result of their indecision, these systems exhibit one or more of the following characteristics, all of which are counterproductive toward achievement of their goals:

- Debates at many levels regarding overall goals and objectives
- Confusion and uncertainty about priorities

FIGURE 3-7. Examples of Systems That Include Provider-owned Health Plans

PPOs

Not-for-Profit Provider-Owned
Baptist Health Services Corporation (Memphis, Tenn.)
Preferred One (Louisville, Ky.)
North Texas Healthcare Network (Irving, Tex.)
Providence Vantage PPO (Portland, Ore.)

For-Profit Provider-Owned
PPO Alliance (Woodland Hills, Calif.)
First Choice Health Network (Bellevue, Wash.)
QualCare Preferred Networks (Piscataway, N.J.)
Sound Health (Seattle, Wash.)

HMOs

Not-for-Profit Provider-Owned
Health Alliance Plan of Michigan (Detroit, Mich.)
Mercy Health Plans (Farmington Hills, Mich.)
Geisinger Health Plan (Danville, Penn.)
Hometown Health Plan–Nevada (Reno, Nev.)

For-Profit Provider-Owned
Partners National Health Plans of Indiana (South Bend, Ind.)
Harris Methodist Texas Health Plan (Arlington, Tex.)
Care America-Southern California (Woodland Hills, Calif.)
Preferred Plus of Kansas (Wichita, Kan.)

Source: Kertesz, L. 1996. Systems begin pruning HMOs from holdings. *Modern Healthcare* 26 (25): 77–86 (17 June).

FIGURE 3-8. Examples of Systems That Have Totally or Partially Divested Themselves of Health Plans

---

Advocate Health Care (Park Ridge, Ill.)
Alternative Health Delivery Systems (Louisville, Ky.)
Dreyer Medical Clinic (Aurora, Ill.)
Graduate Health System (Philadelphia, Penn.)
St. Francis (Pittsburgh, Penn.)

Source: Kertesz, L. 1996. Systems begin pruning HMOs from holdings. *Modern Healthcare* 26 (25): 77–86 (17 June).

- Difficulty making decisions on capital expenditures and resource allocation
- Unrealistic vision and plans
- Impractical arrangements between provider and payer aspects
- Conflicting organizational relationships
- Muddy public image

There is no right or wrong with respect to the combination or separation of health care delivery and financing; much depends on the characteristics of individual markets and organizations. Choosing a course of action, pursuing it, evaluating it, and changing direction if necessary is preferable to avoiding making a decision at all.

Internal Focus

Of the three macro issues in the evolutionary process of system development, internal focus is the most important—and the most difficult. Included in internal focus are functional integration, clinical integration, downsizing and reengineering, leadership, and training and development.

Functional Integration Described in chapter 1, functional integration involves coordination of support functions—for example, human resources, support services, culture, strategic planning, quality assurance, marketing, information systems, and financial management. Although these activities do not need to be centralized to work well, they often are. A common obstacle to functional integration is preexistence within one or more system components of methods that are effective for that component. The need to revise what already works for the sake of the "greater good of the system" is often difficult to accept.

Clinical Integration   Clinical integration, also described in chapter 1, is directed toward the management of individual patients across the continuum of care and the management of the health and wellness of population groups. Payer-driven systems often understand clinical integration better than provider-driven systems. Publicly supported provider-sponsored systems such as state-supported medical centers embrace the concept more easily than private provider-sponsored systems, which frequently have two handicaps: (1) discrepancy between the vision and reality of the continuum of care; and (2) inadequate information systems/ technology.

Continuum of care: Vision versus reality: Many provider-sponsored integrated systems talk about a continuum of care long before they have the pieces in place through ownership and/or contractual relationships. Their language is politically correct, but these systems are not positioned to manage individuals or populations across multiple levels of care.

Case/care management in many provider-sponsored systems illustrates the point. The function has the potential to improve the delivery, management, and coordination of patient care regardless of the settings in which care is provided. In many provider-initiated systems, however, the hospitals developed limited inpatient case management prior to the creation of the system. If the hospitals become part of an integrated system, the inpatient focus of case/care management must be reevaluated so that patients can be managed across the entire system. Frequently, the hospitals stubbornly resist suggestions to modify their existing case management system.

Inadequate information systems/technology: A second obstacle to clinical integration in many provider-driven systems is absence of a patient-focused management information system. In many such systems, information systems architects try to informate the system before the components are in place. In systems initiated and driven by nonproviders, the information systems may have an enrollee focus from the outset.

Downsizing and Reengineering   Downsizing and reengineering often go hand in hand, but they are not synonymous. Downsizing means reduction—in functions, in managerial and supervisory layers, and in staff. Ideally, *after* it has occurred, an integrated system can reevaluate who does what and reengineer appropriately.

Leadership   Leadership is important throughout the process of building integrated health care systems. Different skills are needed at different points in a system's development. Chapter 5 provides details on systems leadership.

Training and Development   Because the concept of integrated health care systems is so new and different in most environments, training and development is an important aspect of internal focus. Board members, senior leadership, middle managers, and staff will all need formal training and ongoing coaching and skill building to help them succeed in their new roles.

GROWTH STAGES

As they mature, systems repeatedly revisit the issues of market, organization, and internal focus. Simultaneously, they experience at least seven stages of growth: preliminary planning, system formation, assimilation, market refocus, acceptance of the importance of the system over its components, redesign, and community health and advocacy (Jones and Mayerhofer 1994). In general, integrated systems must accomplish some activities before moving on to others, but there is usually overlap among the different growth stages. Local market conditions, leadership skills, and many other factors impact the sequence in which the stages occur.

Stage 1: Preliminary Planning

Disparate organizations begin to think of system collaboration when the external environment sends signals. Important events in the legal and regulatory environments often are the catalysts that stimulate coalescence of influence, financial resources, and operational capacity. An example is California: The termination of Hill-Burton funding in 1971, Proposition 13 (which impacted the ability of district and county hospitals to rely on a local tax base), Medi-Cal reform, and the introduction of the diagnosis-related group basis of payment for Medicare all stimulated the growth of systems. In 1996, three different external events promoted still a new round of systems activity. The regulatory stimulus was the expected impact of seismic safety laws on hospital replacement and access to capital. The competitive factor was the anticipation of inroads for for-profit giant Columbia/HCA. Another factor was a change in policy by the state department of corporations and its issuance of a limited HMO license to a provider.

Stage 2: System Formation

Stage two, the formation stage, is the point at which an integrated health care system is legally formed. Organizational structure, governance, and management are put in place. At this stage, many systems are so eager to compete in the marketplace that they abbreviate their deliberations. They neglect the careful development and cultivation of relationships because outright mergers, acquisitions, and similar configurations appear to be the most expeditious ways to rapidly build a system and gain members.

Accelerated systems formation can become problematic if it is not followed by careful attention to operational issues. A good example is the acquisition of physician practices, a strategy often used to strengthen primary care capacity. Many systems rush to close deals to prevent competitors from buying desirable physician practices. When the ink on the agreements dries, however, the day-to-day challenges of managing those practices turn out to be more difficult than anticipated.

At Duke University Medical Center & Health System (see chapter 7), the primary care physician practice acquisition strategy (Duke University Affiliated Physicians, or DUAP) enabled Duke to offer managed care products to university employees and throughout North Carolina. However, the small group of planners who accomplished the practice acquisitions lacked the operational skills needed to manage physicians who were unaccustomed to functioning in a group, let alone in an academic environment. The newly acquired physicians suffered financial losses. To improve the financial situation, Duke Hospital assumed responsibility for daily operations. Unfortunately, the reporting relationship impeded resolution of difficult issues and weakened the overall effectiveness of primary care. The Duke faculty practice plan—the private diagnostic clinic, not Duke Hospital—was the organization with which DUAP physicians and staff needed to integrate.

Another result of accelerated system formation is loss of talented professionals. Many new systems are so eager to reduce operating costs that they immediately lay off many employees. Although that strategy may have short-term financial gains, in the long run, building an integrated system is very complex, and new opportunities may be presented to long-time employees who understand the system and can take on new responsibilities.

Stage 3: Assimilation

At the third stage of growth, many systems begin to replace separate missions, goals, and operations with systems functions. Although assimilation of separate activities could begin earlier, it often does not. The reason is often that concentration on a more integrated structure at an earlier point in time might have been a deal breaker.

When systems assimilate multiple functions into a single system, they usually begin with functional as opposed to clinical integration. For example, they begin with activities such as debt refinancing, insurance, human resources, and the creation of a common system image. Work on information systems/information technology might also start here. Clinical integration is more complex. When it begins, it may be phased in on a service line basis rather than simultaneously for the entire system.

Partners HealthCare System in Boston illustrates the difficulty of assimilation. The system developed from an affiliation of Massachusetts General Hospital and Brigham and Women's Hospital. Systems development occurred relatively quickly once key decision makers at both places had agreed upon this strategy. With equal rapidity, it was announced that for market reasons, each hospital would retain its own name. The consolidation of clinical services, never easy in a single academic medical center—let alone two, was not planned right away (Nessen 1995). In fact, although Brigham and Women's Hospital had a large and excellent maternity service, shortly after the announcement of hospital affiliation and system development, Massachusetts General Hospital went forward with its plans to open its own maternity service. Within a short time, the system's overall market share in obstetrics had increased. Partners' sense of timing was appropriate; tackling clinical integration in a new system might have jeopardized the entire effort. Over time, however, the issue of assimilation must be addressed.

Stage 4: Market Refocus

Having achieved some degree of basic stability by moving through the first three growth stages, systems often pause to reflect and take another serious look at the external market. They revisit the appropriateness of their networks, pricing, internal operations, physician integration, and external relationships. If purchasers in a given market are sophisticated in demands for evidence of quality and cost effectiveness, they may focus on measurable indicators that demonstrate clinical, process, and financial outcomes.

The Kaiser System (Kaiser Foundation Health Plan, Kaiser Foundation Hospitals, and the Permanente Medical Group), an example used repeatedly throughout this book, illustrates market refocus. The Kaiser System has long enjoyed a reputation of success. In the early 1990s, however, enrollment growth was below target, and enrollees were beginning to express preferences for health plans that permitted greater choice of providers and practice settings (Azevedo 1995). In 1991, CalPers, which buys and administers health care for one million California public employees, actually froze enrollment in Kaiser in response to the plan's proposed premium increase.

The event was a sentinel. During the next few years, market-responsive changes included extension of physician participation beyond the traditional staff model to include IPA-type arrangements, reorganization along broad program lines, implementation of many patient-friendly systems improvements, provision of report card–type feedback to employers, merger with another health plan, and consolidation of separate California divisions.

Systems that do not begin with strong physician involvement in governance, leadership, and operations often focus on physician integration at stage 4. The Sisters of Providence Health System in Portland, Ore., owned five hospitals. However, these hospitals and the physicians on their medical staffs were not integrated. To integrate physicians and formalize their leadership role, the system offered a single shareholder opportunity to all physicians.

There is no magic formula for system relationships with health plans. Systems must periodically reevaluate their decisions regarding the integration of health care delivery and financing. Health plan relationships, like provider networks, pricing, customer service, and emphasis on quality, frequently change at the fourth stage of system development. A provider-sponsored system may decide that it needs a "captive plan" and seek out a partner. A system that already has an insurance partner may broaden its relationships with other health plans and even divest itself of its own plan. Or, a system may decide to form its own health plan, even though it has a special relationship with a particular insurer. Medicaid and Medicare managed care opportunities are sometimes the catalyst. In general, most provider-initiated systems do not limit themselves to one option in their health plan relationships.

Stage 5: Acceptance of the Importance of the System over Its Components

In stage 5, turf fights give way to acceptance of the belief that the whole is greater than the sum of its parts. Activities that commonly occur at this stage of growth include attention to culture, strategic planning retreats by boards/senior managers/medical staffs, CQI activities, merging operating and capital budgets, and staff planning across the continuum.

Of all of the activities that occur in the acceptance stage, attention to culture is the one that many of the country's most thoughtful systems executives believe predicts system success or failure. Managing culture change requires mastery of practical strategies and emotional issues. Discussions of vision, values, and new behaviors that can reinforce system mission and goals must come sooner, not later. Yet even if systems directly address the culture issue early in their development, they should expect the change process to last from 3 to 10 years (Kennedy 1996). Table 3-1 identifies system strategies that facilitate or deter cultural change. Four systems that have devoted significant attention to culture changes are Fairview Hospital and Healthcare Services in Minnesota, Centura Health in Colorado, HealthPartners of Southern Arizona, and Henry Ford Health System in Michigan (Kennedy 1996). Case 6-10 includes details about two of these systems.

Stage 6: System Redesign

By stage 6, the previously separate components of an integrated system have intellectually and emotionally accepted the system

TABLE 3-1. Strategies That Facilitate or Derail Postmerger Changes in Culture

	Facilitate	Derail
Timing	Introduce discussion of values, mission, and background during merger planning phase.	Ignore differences; just close deals.
Structure and Systems	Design new structure and systems to facilitate new vision.	Create new name and logo but leave old structures and systems in place.
Speed	Address culture quickly; much else depends on it.	Delay dealing with culture change; it is less tangible than bricks and mortar or other acquisition of assets.
Operational and clinical systems	Redo operational and clinical systems to support new vision.	Allow bigger, richer components of system to dominate.
Relationship of values and behaviors	Link values to behaviors and measure relationships.	Create expectations but no follow-through.
Modeling	Encourage top leaders to act as models.	Ignore impact of behavior of leadership on entire organization.
Rewards	Recognize new culture with understandable and tangible rewards.	Ignore relationship between new values and behaviors and rewards that reinforce them.
Outcomes measurement	Do baseline survey and regular periodic checks.	Ignore value of ongoing measurement.

Source: Kennedy, M. 1996. Creating a new postmerger culture. *Health System Leader* 3 (5): 4–11 (June).

approach. They have accomplished enough as a system so that the external market has reacted to what they have done. They are ready and willing to respond to external needs and demands and, if necessary, make changes. Typically they look at reimbursement, accessibility of care, outcomes, information systems, reorganization of service lines, and creation/revision of internal operating systems.

Reimbursement   Providers may feel confident in system operations and be willing to accept more financial risk or risk sharing. They may alter the way in which dollars are distributed internally to improve alignment of financial incentives. Contract negotiation may be centralized to be more responsive to payer preference.

Accessibility of Care   The provider network designed at the time the system formed may undergo careful scrutiny. It may be expanded and strengthened to provide more accessible care to a more clearly defined geographic area. It may also be more selective within specific specialties. Focus may shift from physicians to alternative caregivers and sites of care.

Quality and Outcomes   Systems have made enough progress with functional and clinical integration to look outward at payer and consumer needs. Quality and outcomes as defined by the market may become a new focus.

Information Systems   As system components are put in place and attention shifts to quality and outcomes, clinical information systems become extremely important. Serious attention may be given to exchanging information throughout the entire continuum of care.

Reorganization of Service Lines   As providers become accustomed to interacting across organizational and facility lines, it may make sense to organize traditional service lines across the continuum of care. Systems that do this must address organization, financial/budget responsibility, information flow, care management, and other complex issues. They often pilot the service line approach slowly, and they may take different approaches for different service lines. The Department of Veterans Affairs, for example, is committed to the service line approach, but different regions will meet the common goal in different ways.

Internal Operating Systems Internal operating systems may be reorganized to focus on patient needs. The service line approach may have a significant impact.

Stage 7: Community Health and Advocacy

Logically, attention to community health and advocacy should guide what systems do and how they do it. But logic does not always prevail. Because of the complexity of creating and developing integrated health care systems, attention is often given to community health and advocacy only after other growth phases. In some systems it may never occur; their major focus may be to reap a financial benefit and not incur the costs of caring for a population of any people other than enrollees. Even for their own members, these systems may not allocate resources to health and wellness.

If and when it occurs, community health and advocacy involves movement away from the events of illness toward the management of health and wellness of both individuals and populations. Techniques by which systems approach that challenge include the following:

- Focus on public health/environment standards
- Disease prevention
- Provision of both medical and social services
- Development of multidisciplinary programs for poverty and aging—for example, nutrition, mental illness, workplace injuries, and exposure to toxic substances

Systems that have concentrated on community health and advocacy include Harvard Pilgrim in New England, Group Health Cooperative of Puget Sound in Washington, Lovelace in New Mexico, and Baptist in Arkansas. Some of these efforts are described in case 6-14. Although integrated health care systems can use community health and advocacy as a competitive advantage, in some places competing systems collaborate for the good of the community at large. Case 6-8 describes examples in Indiana, Texas, and Oregon.

MOVING ALONG

There is no answer to the question, "How long does it take to develop an integrated system?" Each integrated system addresses macro issues and stages of growth in a unique way. Some systems make major and early errors and drop out. Others move slowly, stop to reevaluate their progress, and make changes before moving on. Some systems lay out, follow, and continuously revise long-range plans; most do not.

The case study on Duke University Medical Center & Health System in chapter 7 describes the first stages of building a system. Between 1992 and 1996, Duke aggressively acquired physician practices, developed a joint venture with an insurance company, and accepted full capitation for 35,000 covered lives. However, Duke did not deal with the important issues of clarifying mission and goals, system organization, governance, leadership, and culture change. So the answer to the question regarding length of time to build an integrated system is "a very long time."

References

Azevedo, D. 1995. What you can bargain for when HMOs compete. *Business and Health* 13 (6): 44–56 (June).

Coddington, D. C., C. R. Chapman, and K. M. Pokowski. 1996. *Making integrated health care work: Case studies.* Englewood, Colo.: Center for Research in Ambulatory Health Care Administration.

Ernst & Young, LLP. 1996. *Navigating through the currents.* IDFS Profile. Washington, D.C.: Ernst & Young, LLP.

Flower, J. 1996. Pride and prejudice. *Healthcare Forum Journal* 39 (2): 26–34 (March/April).

Friedman, E. 1996. Too much of a bad thing. *Healthcare Forum Journal* 39 (2):11–15 (March/April).

GHS links regional network of care. 1995. *Health Management Technology* 16 (1): 20–26 (January).

Greene, J., and S. Lutz. 1996. A tale of two ownership sectors. *Modern Healthcare* 26 (2): 61–102 (20 May).

Integrated healthcare 100 directory. 1996. Reston, Va.: St. Anthony Publishing.

Japsen, B. 1996. Survey: Integrated systems pale next to HMOs. *Modern Healthcare* 26 (32): 10 (5 August).

Jones, W. J., and J. J. Mayerhofer. 1994. Regional health care systems: Implications for health care reform. *Managed Care Quarterly* 2 (1): 31–44 (winter).

Kennedy, M. 1996. Creating a new postmerger culture. *Health System Leader* 3 (5): 4–11 (June).

Kertesz, L. 1996. Systems begin pruning HMOs from holdings. *Modern Healthcare* 26 (25): 77–86 (17 June).

Mead-Fox, D., and B. S. Scheur. 1996. Organizational schizophrenia: Provider systems as payers—steps for managing the condition. Presentation at American College of Health Care Executives, 1996 Congress on Healthcare Management, Chicago, 11 March.

Nessen, R. 1995. Presentation at Harvard Conference on Strategic Alliances, Boston, 1–3 November.

Randall, D. A., ed. 1996. *Legal issues and the integrated delivery system: An executive guide.* Chicago: American Hospital Publishing, Inc.

Satinsky, M. A. 1995. *An executive guide to case management strategies.* Chicago: American Hospital Publishing, Inc.

Shortell, S. M., R. R. Gillies, D. A. Anderson, K. M. Erickson, and J. B. Mitchell. 1996. *Remaking health care in America: Building organized delivery systems.* San Francisco: Jossey-Bass.

4

Factors That Contribute to Successful System Integration

INTRODUCTION

Regardless of differences in goals, structure, timetable, and geographic location, integrated health care delivery/financing systems that continue to achieve the goals they set for themselves exhibit many similar qualities. The following attributes have repeatedly been mentioned by researchers who have studied systems, consultants who have facilitated systems formation, and representatives of the systems themselves as contributing to the systems' success:

- Philosophical commitment to the formation and development of integrated health care
- Clarity of purpose and vision
- Physician involvement in key leadership roles
- Alignment of financial incentives and rewards that recognize system performance
- Customer focus
- Information systems and technology that support system goals and operations

- Ongoing emphasis on quality improvement
- Focus on creating market-driven value

This chapter describes each of those attributes, and refers to the cases in chapter 6 to illustrate each point. The variety of examples suggests that no single system is a model for everything. The eight success factors, and several systems that exemplify them, are listed in figure 4-1.

PHILOSOPHICAL COMMITMENT

When different organizations come together to create an integrated health care system, each brings a philosophy that is reflected in individual mission and goals, governance and structure, preferred styles of leadership and decision making, internal and external communications, and organizational culture. Presumably, but not necessarily, the different organizations share a common outlook on many of these factors; otherwise they would have chosen other partners. As a system, the challenge is to build upon what already exists and create a new philosophy that permeates the entire system.

An integrated health care system's formal mission statement and goals are important. Both should reveal what the new organization expects to achieve. Systems that have been initiated by either health plans or providers may identify assumption of responsibility for the health and wellness of both individuals and target populations as their top priority. Systems with religious origins/sponsorship may articulate commitment to care for all people, regardless of ability to pay. Other systems may be less interested in the health and wellness of defined populations than they are in acquisition, growth, and expansion; their mission statements emphasize strong financial performance. Systems connected with academic medical centers may include educational and research components in their missions. Finally, systems that include both provider and financing components may identify multiple missions and goals that require a delicate balance.

After integrated health care systems have legally been formed, governance, like mission and goals, reflects philosophical commitment to build a system. When different organizations join forces to form a system, system board members may continue to represent

FIGURE 4-1. Success Factors as Exemplified by Specific Integrated Systems

Success Factor	Systems with Proven Track Records
Philosophical commitment to systems integration	Advocate Health Care (Illinois); Henry Ford Health System (Michigan)
Clarity of purpose and vision	Baylor Health Care System (Texas); Copley Health System (Vermont)
Strong physician leadership	Fairview Hospital and Healthcare Services (Minnesota); Friendly Hills HealthCare Network (California); Henry Ford Health System (Michigan); North Shore Medical Center (Massachusetts)
Alignment of financial incentives and rewards that recognized system performance	Samaritan Health System (Arizona)
Customer focus on purchasers; enrollees; system components; legal, regulatory, and accrediting agencies; and communities	Appalachian Regional Healthcare (Kentucky, Virginia, West Virginia); Carolinas HealthCare System (North and South Carolina); Group Health Cooperative (Washington); Laurel Health System (Pennsylvania)
Information systems and technology that support systems goals and operations	Advocate Health Care (Illinois); Allina Health System (Minnesota); Graduate Health System (New Jersey, Pennsylvania)
Ongoing emphasis on quality improvement	Harvard Pilgrim Health Care (New England); Henry Ford Health System (Michigan); Lovelace Health Systems (New Mexico); Presbyterian Healthcare Services (New Mexico)
Focus on creating market-driven value	Dartmouth-Hitchcock Health System—Northern Region (New England); Henry Ford Health System (Michigan); Mercy Health Services (Michigan)

the separate constituencies from which they came, rather than the new system. One way to avoid this dilemma is to exclude existing board members from participation in system governance. A more moderate approach that helps systems build upon the strengths of their founding organizations while moving forward is to allow previous board members to join the system board, but to quickly focus that new board on development of the system mission and goals. Another technique for facilitating system governance is system education for all board members, regardless of their previous experiences in governance.

Formal statements of missions, goals, and governance are just the beginning. Philosophical commitment to building a system then impacts leadership and decision making. In one system that is the product of a merger of two previously successful systems, operational leaders in different delivery sites also assume corporate responsibilities for system activities.

Internal and external communications can reinforce philosophical commitment to building an integrated health care system. Systems executives can share systems priorities not only with people working within the system but also with those who are outside it and in a position to direct business toward or away from it. Senior leadership can be honest about the challenges of making systems work, and they can encourage staff to make difficult but necessary professional and personal adjustments. Systems can reward both individuals and teams for their contributions to system successes.

Even when a system philosophy exists, participants may have difficulty relinquishing old styles and learning new ways of relating to each other. The key to ensuring that day-to-day functions are consistent with the corporate mission includes identifying differences in culture among system components, developing a plan to create a new system culture, and carefully nurturing that implementation.

The Henry Ford Health System in Michigan has articulated and operationalized its philosophical commitment to building an integrated system (case 6-9). It also continues to develop its system culture (case 6-10).

CLARITY OF PURPOSE AND VISION

Successful integrated health care systems are clear about purpose and vision. They arrive at consensus through formal planning processes that enable them to (1) accumulate and analyze information; (2) involve operational managers in future thinking; (3) critically discuss goals, strategy, and resources; (4) link short-term activities to long-term plans; and (5) generate special studies on important issues (Bennis and Nanus 1985). Systems that take the time to work through their missions, goals, priorities, and related operations are the most likely to mobilize their organizations to achieve desired results.

Kongstvedt and Gates of Ernst & Young suggest that integrated health care systems must deal with at least the following strategic issues during their planning processes: preservation and expansion of patient base; control; maintenance versus shifting of income for system components; special programs/missions such as teaching; quality; and downsizing/jobs (Kongstvedt and Gates 1996). In addition, another aspect of integrated systems that must be planned is the process itself. Many systems ignore the point completely; they initiate multiple unrelated projects and let them evolve.

These suggestions appear straightforward. Yet obstacles often prevent systems from clarifying purpose and vision through formalized planning. First, many integrated systems are guided by a strong leader or small group of people who have been willing to take the risks necessary to initiate the change process. Often these key players lack the interest in and patience for the methodical and time-consuming planning that must be done during the early development stages. The integrated system scatters its human and financial resources in many different directions.

A second obstacle to clarification of system purpose and vision is resistance to the concept of an integrated system. Each system component may already have an internal planning process, but if systemwide planning does not occur before or shortly after the system's legal formation, the system will evolve without a road map and probably continue along an ill-defined course.

Academic medical centers involved in developing integrated systems face a third obstacle to clarification of purpose and vision. Many aggressively market their new system status but leave existing organizational structures intact. Despite what the billboards advertise, the separate components of the system continue to make their own plans, but those components compete rather than collaborate with each other.

In spite of these potential obstacles, some systems have taken the time to plan their courses of action in both short- and long-term time frames. Examples include Baylor Health Care System in Texas and Copley Health System in rural Vermont (case 6-11).

PHYSICIAN INVOLVEMENT IN KEY LEADERSHIP ROLES

Some of the more successful integrated systems in the country originated in physician group practices or foundations for medical care. Lovelace Health Systems in New Mexico, Mayo Clinic in Minnesota, Kaiser in multiple locations, Cleveland Clinic in Ohio, and Geisinger Health System in Pennsylvania are among them. However, many of the newer integrated systems have had different origins; they have been founded by hospitals, hospital networks, health plans, insurance companies, or combinations thereof. As a result, these newer entities with nonphysician sponsorship have not always started with strong physician leadership. The more successful ones have quickly discovered that strong physician leadership and integration of physicians into the total system are essential. Examples of integrated systems that recognize the importance of physician leadership and demonstrate that commitment are described in case 6-12: the Henry Ford Health System in Michigan, Fairview Hospital and Healthcare Services in Minnesota, Friendly Hills HealthCare Network in California, and North Shore Health System in Massachusetts.

Important Concepts

Physician integration and strong leadership involve at least the following five components:

- Emphasis on management of care by primary care practitioners
- Physician representation in governance and administration
- Physician involvement in operations, particularly care management across the continuum
- Physician acceptance of financial risk and alignment of physician and system financial incentives
- Education and training for physicians that focuses on management of care, cost and quality, and leadership skills

Management of Care by Primary Care Practitioners
Regardless of the system's sponsorship, primary care is important to all integrated health care systems. Without an adequate supply and geographic distribution of primary care providers, a system cannot

attract a sufficient number of enrollees, manage health and wellness, meet patient expectations, and retain and gain membership.

Adequate primary care capacity does not work miracles if other caregivers in the system, as well as the enrollees, do not understand and accept the role of primary care. It is imperative that primary care providers and specialists clarify the role that each will play in the provision and coordination of patient care. They can do this by jointly reviewing/developing clinical practice guidelines and by agreeing on appropriate responsibilities for diagnosis, consultation, treatment, and follow-up. They can also encourage their office staffs, who will be coordinating referrals and follow-up, to develop administrative procedures that support the role of primary care providers. If primary care providers and their staffs are clear about their roles, they can give a clear and consistent message to enrollees and to other clinicians. When they are unclear, enrollees become caught up in internal confusion, feel as if they are being short-changed, and often become dissatisfied with the entire system.

Physician Representation in Governance and Administration   Physician representation in governance and administration also is important. Group practices, foundations, and more recently IPAs and PHOs have afforded physicians good opportunities to lead and participate in both governance and administration. However, many other health care organizations have historically limited physician board participation and involvement in daily operations.

For example, in the acute hospital world, physicians typically have had token representation on hospital boards and exercised their influence through medical staff channels. A medical director position has existed in some but not all places. Between 1993 and 1996, the Internal Revenue Service (IRS) limited physician representation on the boards of integrated delivery systems to 20 percent. A new policy has raised the limit to 49 percent, provided that physicians comply with strict rules governing conflict of interest (Greene 1996).

Physician Involvement in Operations   Management of care across the continuum clearly requires physician direction and cooperation. Corporate mergers, acquisitions, and technologies such as telemedicine cannot improve patient care if physicians cannot or will not collaborate. Furthermore, in a managed care environment, physicians not only must manage care; they also must be able to demonstrate quality of clinical, financial, and process outcomes.

Physician Acceptance of Financial Risk Physician acceptance of financial risk for the cost and utilization of patient care and the linkage of physician and system financial incentives is imperative. If physicians' financial incentives differ from those of other system components, or if physicians in different specialties have inconsistent financial incentives, they will not be motivated to focus on the goals of the total system.

Physician Education and Training Finally, physicians in key leadership roles can be more effective if their clinical training is supplemented with skill development in areas such as communication, leadership skills, team building, negotiation and conflict resolution, and quality management (Leider and Bard 1994).

Barriers to Physician Involvement

Both external and internal barriers impede systems' attempts to ensure physician involvement in key leadership roles (Shortell and others 1996). Externally, the U.S. health care system has remained a crazy quilt; provider reimbursement has continued to vary by payer, sending confusing messages to potential future leaders. Large public programs such as Medicare and Medicaid, with separate reimbursement mechanisms for hospitals and physicians, have reinforced the problem. As already mentioned, from 1993 to 1996, IRS restrictions limited physician representation on the boards of integrated systems. Faced with inconsistent and shifting financial incentives, many physicians focus solely on their practices rather than on leadership. Internally, physicians do not assume leadership roles in systems activities because of unwillingness to accept the reality of a changing marketplace. Further, fear, lack of information, and inexperience in governance and managerial roles hold them back.

Inducements for Physician Involvement

Just as external and internal barriers discourage physician involvement in key leadership roles in integrated systems, other external and internal factors encourage physician involvement. Some of these are dissatisfaction with the status quo and determination to help shape their own destiny; understanding of and commitment to system vision; empowerment through skill building; and availability of internal support systems such as management information and a strong CQI process.

ALIGNMENT OF FINANCIAL INCENTIVES AND REWARDS

All integrated health care systems must align financial incentives and rewards to recognize system performance. If financial arrangements are inconsistent with system long-term goals or if financial incentives are mixed within a given system, progress and success will be negatively affected.

Three concepts are important, and systems must address all of them: (1) willingness to accept financial risk for the cost and utilization of care; (2) consistency of financial incentives; and (3) financial rewards for system performance.

Willingness to Accept Financial Risk

Willingness to accept financial risk for the cost and utilization of care means that health care providers (as well as the insurer if the integrated entity includes financing) agree to accept financial responsibility and accountability for the health care that is delivered. Providers and/or insurers are willing to operate within a limited budget; if either the cost or the utilization of care exceeds expectations, they are penalized financially.

Consistency of Financial Incentives

Existence of consistent financial incentives throughout the system means that different participants in the system have consistent, although not necessarily identical, financial incentives. For example, a system may include primary care providers, specialists, acute hospitals, home care, alternative care, and other components. It will certainly include clinical, administrative, and support people. The system may own some but not all of its components. Financial incentives for all components and people must recognize and reward the same behaviors. Desirable clinical outcomes and processes must be clear to all.

Financial Rewards for System Performance

Creation of financial rewards that recognize system performance is the third important concept. Systems that address this particular issue often learn this challenge is not only about money; it is about system culture and values. In so many systems, the components that comprise them have historically been reactive organizations. Structures and decision making have been hierarchical, and collaboration has been the exception, not the norm. Most have provided care to sick people who have presented with symptoms. When systems revise their values and culture, they embrace different principles: proactive behavior, flattened decision making, teamwork with other system components and with external agencies, and focus on keeping enrollees well. New compensation models must reward these new ideas (Moore 1996).

One of the reasons that systems have had difficulty relating compensation to system performance is that system mission, goals, and values are not always clear. Nonetheless, some systems have done a good job at aligning incentives. Case 6-13 describes Phoenix-based Samaritan Health System's rewards for employee behaviors that support the system.

Another problem for many systems is that they address some but not all three components of alignment of incentives and appropriate rewards. Systems may negotiate capitation contracts but neglect the two other pieces—making rewards throughout the system consistent with one another, and rewarding behaviors that support system goals.

CUSTOMER FOCUS

Market-sensitive integrated systems know that the legal act of creating a system and early decisions on governance and management do not guarantee success. Of greater importance is the system's ability to look outside itself into the marketplace and to respond to the expectations of multiple customers. Some of these expectations are clearly articulated; others are more subtle.

Just who are a system's customers? There are at least four answers: purchasers, enrollees, system components, and external customers. The needs of the four different groups are not always in harmony, making effective response a delicate balancing act.

Purchasers as Customers

Purchasers include private and public employers and formal health care purchasing groups that represent employers. They regularly evaluate/reevaluate their options for health insurance. As customers of integrated systems, purchasers articulate their expectation in a variety of ways. They may insist on specific methods and amounts of reimbursement. They may limit the dollars they are willing to pay for annual premiums or premium increases, and they may require providers to assume a certain degree of financial risk. Because purchasers buy on behalf of specific populations, they may also identify desirable health outcomes and targets for quality improvement.

Purchasing groups in California and Minnesota exemplify the ways in which purchasers as customers can impact integrated systems. The Pacific Business Group on Health (PBGH), based in San Francisco, is a not-for-profit coalition of public and private purchasers. Collectively, PBGH members spend $3 million annually on health care. The group was formed in 1994 to negotiate both price and quality with California HMOs. In summer 1996, PBGH announced that 15 HMOs providing care to 500,000 public and private employees and to 40,000 Medicare-eligible retirees had agreed to keep 1997 premium levels flat. At the same time, the group outlined several quality initiatives (California purchasing co-op 1996).

The Minneapolis–St. Paul Buyers Healthcare Action Group (BHCAG) is a midwestern purchasing group with system customers. By 1996, BHCAG represented 23 employers, including most of the large private groups and the state of Minnesota. It offered members a common self-insured point-of-service plan and contracted with a limited number of integrated systems and 50 medical groups (Kemnitz 1996). Future plans called for competitive bidding by health care teams. BHCAG has been influential, and each of the systems and groups with which it relates has tried to accommodate to its changing needs.

Enrollees as Customers

Enrollees are also customers of integrated health care systems. They can choose from among the options offered by purchasers. Enrollee expectations vary with buyer sophistication. Some enrollees are knowledgeable and assertive health care purchasers. Others who are less well informed express their expectations in negative ways—by complaints or retrospectively through the grievance process.

More informed enrollees ask many questions about systems before selecting a health insurance plan. They look at factors such as benefit coverage, monthly premiums, co-payments, provider network, clinical reputation, and health plan policies and procedures for referrals. After enrollment, all of these factors remain important, but the reality of receiving care from a health system then sets in. Availability of appointments, provider responsiveness to questions, and actual (as opposed to theoretical) ease of referrals become important to enrollees when they access the health care system. Most important to enrollees is clinical integration. Although enrollees do not use that term, if the system does not look and function like a system, the enrollee will choose another option.

System Components as Customers

Integrated systems are complex organizations. Regardless whether the system components are connected by common ownership, contractual relationships, loose affiliations, or a combination of methods, those components will have multiple and not always identical expectations regarding missions, goals, priorities, accountability, and autonomy. If the different parts of the same system do not hear and respond to each other's needs, the system will not live up to its potential.

Many systems that were not initiated by physicians have difficulty integrating physicians into their decision-making and operational processes. Commonly, such systems emphasize growth of the provider base by offering physicians multiple options for system participation (for example, practice acquisition, contractual relationships, or administrative services). If the strategy is appealing and physicians become part of the system, the system must then respond to the many needs and concerns of individual physicians, small groups, and large groups. All are physician customers within the system itself.

Two California examples illustrate the challenge of responding to physicians as customers in a systems context. Friendly Hills HealthCare Network in California has had a long-standing reputation as a successful integrated delivery system. By the end of 1995, Friendly Hills had 100,000 enrollees. In January 1996, that enrollment had grown to 400,000, when Caremark International, Inc., then the parent of Friendly Hills, purchased practices previously owned by CIGNA. A major system challenge was to make sure that the physicians from the original Friendly Hills Medical Group and the CIGNA physicians shared governance and operational responsibility and pursued common goals (Friendly Hills 1996).

PacifiCare Health Systems, Inc., in Cypress, Calif., is another example of system response to its own physicians as customers. The results of system market research indicated that physicians as well as members were dissatisfied with the existing requirements for specialist referral. To improve the situation, the system initiated a phased statewide change to streamline specialist referrals. A policy that required primary care physician and system medical director/ utilization review committee approval of all referrals was modified (Member complaints 1996).

External Customers

The accountability of integrated health care systems to external customers comprises three components: (1) clinicians, employers, and patients outside the system who refer to it; (2) regulatory and licensing bodies; and (3) communities. System accountability to external customers is evolving.

Most systems are not totally self-contained and depend on referrals from outside the system. The referrals may come from clinicians, employers, and patients themselves. Systems must therefore pay close attention to access, treatment, follow-up, and resolution of complaints for each of these different constituencies.

The concept of integration in the health care field is relatively new. Federal, state, and local regulatory and licensing bodies have not uniformly decided if, when, or how to respond. At times a legal challenge calls the question. For example, in 1994, Blue Cross & Blue Shield of Wisconsin, which owned an HMO called Compcare, sued the Marshfield Clinic for illegally building a monopoly in large parts of the state by forcing physicians to sign exclusive contracts with it. Ultimately, the U.S. Court of Appeals in Chicago reversed an earlier decision against the clinic, ruling that Marshfield is not an illegal monopoly. The decision reaffirmed the clinic's position that an integrated system is best suited for rural health care delivery (Marshfield Clinic 1995).

The overall question of system regulation in the future remains unanswered. In the short run, the components of which systems are made (for example, the delivery system and/or a health plan component) remain accountable to those agencies to which they have historically answered. For example, hospitals that are a part of integrated systems have continued to seek Joint Commission accreditation. Managed care plans that are part of systems continue to meet federal and state requirements and to seek accreditation from the NCQA.

Health care organizations and the insurance industry are accustomed to responding to regulatory requirements. Both have been less consistent in responding to what might be regarded as the *ultimate external customer, the community*. More and more integrated systems have discovered the potential symbiosis between integrated health care delivery/financing and healthy communities. This realization has resulted from multiple trends.

The public health sector has always focused on community health. Health status assessment, programs targeted at particular health risks and problems, and health education and wellness have been cornerstones of the public health movement (McBride 1996). In the managed care industry, the financial structure of HMOs has long been based upon each plan's assumption of responsibility for the health and wellness of a defined enrollee population. The advent of HMO credentialing by the NCQA and the use of HEDIS indicators for evaluating health plans have strengthened the concept of accountability for a population.

More recently, the American Hospital Association and the Healthcare Forum have promoted healthier communities (American Hospital Association 1993; Mudd 1996). The premise of both efforts is that collaboration will improve a community's health status through the provision of a seamless continuum of services by health care providers who are operating within a fixed budget and are accountable to the community. Financial support for these efforts has come from the W. K. Kellogg Foundation, The Duke Endowment, the Catholic Health Association, Voluntary Hospitals of America, and the Hospital Research and Educational Trust.

Finally, managed care plans and public health agencies have discovered that they have much in common. The polarity between them is dissipating, giving way to a variety of structural, functional, and strategic models for interaction (Halverson, Mays, Kaluzny, and Richards 1997).

Many, but not all, integrated health care systems are clear about their ultimate responsibility to defined communities. Yet, even in systems where community health is a priority, the term "community" has a variety of meanings. "Community" may mean individual enrollees who have selected the system and who technically belong to it. It may also mean the community at large, including, but not limited to, system enrollees. Some systems have gone one step further and articulated an obligation to provide care not only for those enrollees who technically belong to them and for whom they collect premiums, but also for people who cannot afford to pay.

Although the long-term benefits from systems that focus on healthier communities have not yet been proven, there are good examples of systems efforts. Case 6-14 describes Group Health Cooperative in Washington, Laurel Health System in Pennsylvania, and Appalachian Regional Healthcare in Kentucky, Virginia, and West Virginia. The profile of Carolinas HealthCare System in case 6-2 describes a unique partnership between the system and a county health department.

INFORMATION SYSTEMS AND TECHNOLOGY THAT SUPPORT SYSTEM GOALS AND OPERATIONS

Information systems/information technology (IS/IT) is the gas that fuels the systems engine; with no fuel or with the wrong kind of fuel, that engine will not run. By contrast, when information systems and technology support a system, and when information is used appropriately, clinicians, enrollees, and external purchasers all benefit.

Important applications of IS/IT in integrated health care systems include systemwide appointment scheduling, electronic medical records, medical work stations, "smart cards" that enrollees carry with them, on-line consultation, telemedicine, and voice recognition (Gates 1996).

The Challenge

The IS/IT challenge facing integrated health care systems is complex for five reasons: (1) the speed of technological change; (2) the interdependence of IS/IT and system mission and goals; (3) the necessity for customization; (4) the importance of careful planning as well as implementation; and (5) the common presumption that IS/IT is a solution, not a support function.

Speed of Technological Change   The technological aspects of the informating task are daunting. Technology will continue to change rapidly. On one hand, systems that wait for the perfect solution will lag behind the competition. On the other hand, those that recommend large capital expenditures may inadvertently limit their future ability to adapt to technological change on a timely basis.

Interdependence of IS/IT and System Mission and Goals   A second aspect of the IS/IT challenge in integrated systems is the interdependence of IS/IT goals and the overall system mission and goals. If an integrated system lacks a clear mission, purpose, and priorities, informating its parts will be more difficult. Nevertheless, that limitation has not deterred many systems from prematurely laying off information systems staff and hastily spending millions of dollars on new technology.

Necessity for Customization   A third aspect of the IS/IT challenge is the need to customize. Every integrated system is unique in history, mission, structure, and operations. It is probable that some IS/IT capability (for example, legacy system) already exists when each system begins. Systems leaders should evaluate a variety of options, including but by no means limited to starting over, modifying preexisting IS/IT components, and combining both options.

Although a number of integrated systems have made good progress in informating themselves, there still is no perfect system. In each example described in case 6-15, the IS/IT approach has been tailored to suit the system, the culture, and the long-term strategy. The examples are Advocate Health Care in Illinois, Allina Health System in Minnesota, and Graduate Health System in Pennsylvania.

Importance of Planning   A fourth challenge in building effective IS/IT is the challenge of process. IS/IT goes beyond technology; it is about people. Although many systems look to their chief information officers (CIOs) to guide them in planning for IS/IT, many CIOs have only operational experience and are not prepared for the complex planning that must take place. Clinicians and organizations that are fighting to protect their turf often dominate the discussions. All too often, the process moves out of control.

Erroneous Presumption that IS/IT Is a Solution

Finally, many integrated health care systems erroneously presume that IS/IT is a solution rather than a means to accomplishing other goals (Van Etten 1996). This prevailing mythology creates a major impediment to progress. IS/IT must support an integrated system so that it can accomplish its goals.

Important Factors

Although the obstacles to informating integrated systems are formidable, systems that are well along in their efforts have learned important lessons and have been willing to share their experiences. Important points are (1) clarity of system and IS/IT purposes; (2) focus on essential elements; (3) logical sequencing; and (4) clinician input and leadership (Reep 1995; Glaser 1995; Gates 1996).

Clarity of System and IS/IT Purposes   As chapter 1 explains, the term *integrated health care delivery/financing system* has multiple meanings. Sometimes, but not always, health care financing and delivery come together in a single system. Sometimes integration is horizontal among like entities; sometimes it is vertical among unlike entities within the health delivery system or between the delivery system and a health plan. Within an integrated system, functional, clinical, virtual, and visual integration are important.

When integrated health care systems are clear in overall mission, goals, and priorities, the IS/IT system design and implementation has the potential to support the entire system. Figure 4-2 illustrates the following potential functions that IS/IT might support in an integrated system that combines both health care delivery and financing:

- Provider network development
- Care management
- Health plan sales and marketing

FIGURE 4-2.   Functions Potentially Supported by IS/IT in an Integrated System

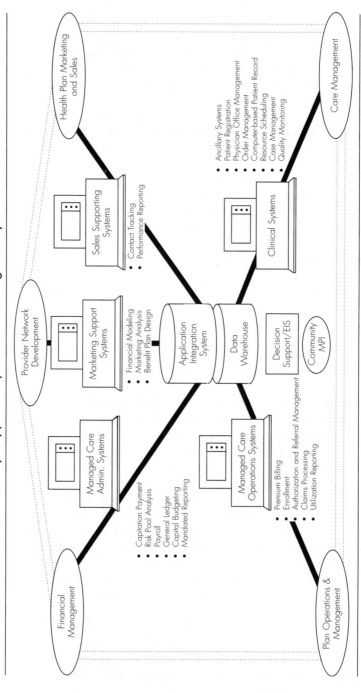

Source: Reep, J. 1995. Integrated Healthcare Report, presented at Integrated Healthcare Symposium, Aspen, Colo., 25–26 September.

- Health plan operations and management
- Financial management

If an integrated system includes the delivery but not the financing of care, the IS/IT will be more limited in scope. For example, it does not need to support health plan enrollment and claims processing. However, it does need to assist the delivery system to manage both care and dollars in a risk-bearing situation.

Focus on Essential Elements CIOs and consultants who have worked with them have generally agreed that IS/IT in integrated systems needs four basic elements: (1) an application integration engine; (2) master patient index; (3) common definitions of terms; and (4) accessible data repository(ies) (Gates 1996).

Application integration engine: When integrated systems form, their components are likely to have a variety of different computer applications that speak different languages and do not connect with one another. For example, encounter-based clinical and financial information may reside in separate systems. Because of historical fee-for-service reimbursement, clinical information may be specific to a delivery site—for example, inpatient, outpatient, home care, long-term care, laboratory, radiology, and pharmacy. Claims-based information that is available from both private and public insurers may not connect with information that has been generated internally.

The application integration engine links different systems within and across organizations. One way in which connections can be made is through distributed client/server computing. With this type of architecture, multiple computer terminals can be distributed throughout the system and connected to one or more servers and each other through a network. The operating system, applications, software, and data are stored on various servers but are accessible throughout the network (Glossary 1996).

Master patient index: If integrated systems focus on meeting patient needs, they need the capability to collect information on individual patients/enrollees, regardless of where and when care is delivered. The concept of patient-specific information is different from that of care-specific collection of information that is currently the norm. Now, for example, within an acute care setting, patient registration systems exist for the convenience of scheduling and billing staff. Inpatient and outpatient medical records may be separate. Results of ancillary testing may be housed departmentally. Information on mental health and substance abuse care may also be detached. Outside the acute care setting, there is often no easy way to obtain information from other sites where care was delivered.

With a patient-specific master index, each patient or member of a system is assigned a single access code, often his or her Social Security number. Clinical and financial information from multiple sources is entered into a single system by using the patient-specific identifier. The method for information entry works regardless of where care has been delivered.

Common definitions of terms: If entries to a patient-specific master index can be made from multiple points in the system, agreement on common language and standard definitions is important. As integrated systems evolve, they must update the common dictionary on an ongoing basis.

Accessible data repository(ies): If clinical and financial information on individual patients/members is entered in a common language, the next step is to keep it in one or more repositories that can be accessed to support a variety of system functions. Clinicians can use it to review historical information on patient illness and treatment. Schedulers can determine whether or not prior authorization and precertification have been completed. Financial staff can call up billing information. Most important in a systems context, caregivers at any place in the system can follow patients across multiple sites and get real-time feedback on problems, test results, and treatment—information they can use to improve their coordination and management of patient care.

Accessibility of patient-specific information housed in one or more common repositories does not obviate the need for appropriate confidentiality. Some ways in which precautions can be taken include testing security controls prior to systemwide installation, making different levels of data available to designated users, and using temporary patient aliases if necessary (Protecting patient confidentiality 1996).

Logical Sequencing   If systems use their IS/IT capabilities to facilitate achievement of strategic goals, they must carefully plan the order of the steps they take. Believing that many systems waste dollars and talent by presuming that they must immediately replace all existing systems with new technology, experienced CIOs recommend the following:

- Completion of IS/IT planning *prior* to making major decisions about technology and staff.
- Coordination of IS/IT planning and implementation with system planning. Sophisticated technology must complement the system configuration.

Clinician Input and Leadership   Clinicians in leadership positions are the ultimate users of information and the most important members of any team that evaluates options and makes decisions for IS/IT. Those who understand the direction of the entire integrated system are also important team members. Many integrated systems, however, automatically expect their CIOs to lead the process of planning and implementing IS/IT. From the perspective of the CIOs themselves, they often feel more comfortable as technical consultants, not as leaders of the decision-making process.

ONGOING EMPHASIS ON QUALITY IMPROVEMENT

Attention to quality is an imperative for integrated health care systems. Although a small number of systems stand out for their accomplishments (case 6-16), relatively few systems are proficient in defining quality, measuring it, and using the results to make changes that have a demonstrable, positive impact on the health status of individuals and populations.

The challenge of quality in a systems context involves conceptualization, technical competence, and, most important, the ability to apply the results to methods for improvement. That challenge entails five key issues: (1) consensus on definitions; (2) acceptance of the importance of quality in helping a system provide better patient care and achieve its goals; (3) application of quality standards to the entire system; (4) mastery of techniques for measurement, documentation, and reporting quality; and (5) development of mechanisms for quality improvement.

Consensus on Definitions

Although the quality of health care receives a great deal of attention, it is a confusing subject. As pointed out in the series of articles on quality that appeared in the *New England Journal of Medicine* in 1996, earlier notions of quality were relatively straightforward (Berwick 1996; Blumenthal 1996a, 1996b; Blumenthal and Epstein 1996; Brook, McGlynn, and Cleary 1996; Chassin 1996). Historically, physicians defined the technical quality of care. Two things were important: the appropriateness of the services provided, and the skill with which care was performed. Quality meant doing the right thing in the right way (Blumenthal 1996).

Over the years, the concept of quality in health care has changed to include quality assessment, quality assurance, TQM, and CQI, a component of TQM. Many integrated health care systems do not clearly understand their distinctions.

Quality assessment means measurement of the level of quality at a particular point in time. It involves comparing professional performance with respect to patient, administrative, and support services against preestablished standards. Limited to problem identification, it does not involve action to improve problem areas (Fazen 1994).

Quality assurance includes but is not limited to quality assessment. It implies that problem areas can not only be identified but also corrected through quality improvement efforts. In hospitals, quality assurance activities have been closely associated with the interests of third-party payers, particularly HCFA, and accreditation agencies such as the Joint Commission. To qualify for reimbursement and accreditation, organizations have developed both departmental and institutionwide quality assurance programs that help them meet the external standards that have been set for them. Managed care organizations also have developed quality assurance programs to review provider practice patterns and utilization and to ensure that maintenance of quality is not compromised by activities directed toward cost control.

New approaches to quality in health care, such as *TQM* and *CQI,* borrow heavily from industry. Instead of focusing negatively on crises and the failure of individuals to conform to standards set by experts, they work positively toward engaging everyone within an organization in ongoing work to raise the overall performance level (Kongstvedt 1993). The process of identifying goals, setting standards, evaluating performance against benchmarks, identifying problems, taking corrective action, and making ongoing improvements is cyclical and unending. Quality applies to an entire organization rather than to separate components. Because the quality improvement process is never finished, individuals within that organization are repeatedly asked to participate on teams that search for ways to do better.

The TQM philosophy changed the definition of quality in another important way. The ultimate goal of TQM and the activities it comprises is to meet or exceed customer expectations. No longer is quality defined only by health care providers. The values and opinions of the consumers of care and of those who pay for care are now part of the quality equation. For example, consumers care about appropriateness of care and clinical excellence, but they also care about access to care, convenience, receipt of timely feedback, and coordination of care across multiple sites. When consumers are asked to evaluate their experience with a health care system, they often describe these processes, not technical competence of physicians or clinical outcomes. Purchasers of care also have something to say about quality.

Chapter 2 describes some of the ways in which employers and purchasing groups express their expectations and measure quality. Some key questions for purchasers include the following (Darling 1995):

- Are they getting what they think they are paying for?
- Are they paying for what they want?
- Is the health care delivery system delivering what it thinks it is?
- Is the health care system/plan delivering what it wants to deliver?
- Is the health care system/plan producing services in the most efficient and effective ways?
- Is the health care system/plan providing services in a way that is superior to those of other similarly positioned systems/plans with similar populations?
- How does the health system/plan compare against benchmarks?
- What changes need to be made to improve performance in each area?

If integrated health care systems are serious about quality, they must develop consensus on definition so that the term is understood both internally and externally. In so doing, they must blend multiple expectations into a coherent concept that works for them.

Acceptance of the Importance of Quality

Once integrated health care systems agree on a definition of quality, they must deal with another issue: Why bother about quality at all? Not everyone supports the expanded definition of quality in health care, and there are strong critics both inside and outside the health care system. For example, physicians often dismiss the input of nonphysicians as to the definition of quality (Chassin 1996). Other health care professionals are uncomfortable with the role that consumers, health plans, and employers now play in articulating their expectations of quality. Skeptics contend that quality means compliance with requirements set by agencies and organizations outside the health care system. They believe that quality parameters are poorly disguised marketing ploys directed toward cost reduction. They are mistrustful of the validity of information that is presented in report cards, and they have serious doubts about the relationship between quality and patient care. They remain closed-minded about the potential value of quality and about their own involvement.

Outside the health care delivery system, health care quality receives attention in two ways. Employers, purchasing coalitions, and other groups that are systematically measuring quality are willing and eager to share their information in the media. At both state and federal levels, there is growing interest in protecting the quality of health care by prohibiting specific health plan reimbursement practices. However, many of these critics of health care quality have not demonstrated their commitment to ensuring it by offering financial support, either through increased reimbursement or direct support for quality activities.

Integrated health care systems that understand the potential of quality in the broad sense are neither suspicious of its importance nor reticent to commit financial resources to make it happen. They embrace it positively in much the same way that non-health-care companies pride themselves on the quality of the products or services they produce or provide. These systems use the quality imperative as a powerful means to improve patient care by reducing unwanted variation. Quality inspires them to excellence that meets both internal and external expectations.

Application of Quality Standards to the Entire System

As described in chapter 3, integrated systems evolve over time, and the process is likely to take many years to complete. As systems evolve, components and relationships repeatedly change. It is indeed difficult to conceptualize and implement a quality program for a large and complex organization that does not remain in one place for long.

Nonetheless, quality should not wait until an integrated system is finished. It must be defined and activated during the early stages of development, and revised and fine-tuned as the system grows.

Mastery of Techniques for Measuring, Documenting, and Reporting Quality

The technical challenge surrounding quality in an integrated health care system is daunting. The state-of-the-art system requires a clear focus on measurement, documentation, and reporting, as well as attention to coordination of all these efforts.

What to Measure? Although the meaning of health care quality in the 1990s is much broader than it was formerly, structure, process, and outcomes remain the focus of quality measurement (Donabedian 1982). Each of these factors (or combinations of them) impact the functions of integrated systems: prevention and screening, access to care, disease management, provision of health care treatments and procedures, management of enrollees' health, and management of the health of populations (fig. 4-3). Quality indicators can measure each cell in the matrix.

Structure: Structure in an integrated system means the fixed ways in which the system components are organized and relate to one another. Ownership, affiliation, daily operations, and capacity are aspects of structure. Although structure is generally measured in descriptive ways, it can have a significant impact on the processes and outcomes of care. For example, if a system's mammography center is located at a site that is inconvenient for patients, the percentage of women who have mammograms will be below the standard. As a result, the incidences of breast cancer beyond stage 1 and mortality rates may be higher than desirable because of a structural feature (Cutler 1995).

FIGURE 4-3.   Quality in Integrated Health Care Systems

The following matrix offers a basic guide to systems in their ongoing assessment of quality. For each matrix cell, a system can frame relevant questions, develop methods to evaluate current status, and, based on the results of the measurements, modify its current state to achieve more desirable results. Several sample questions follow the matrix.

	Access to Care	Prevention and Screening	Disease Management	Treatment and Procedures	Management of Enrollee Health	Management of Health of Populations
Structure	A	B	C	D	E	F
Process	G	H	I	J	K	L
Outcome	M	N	O	P	Q	R

Sample Questions

G.   Process/Access to Care

Do the system's processes enable enrollees/members/patients to access advice and treatment when they need and want it? If not, what barriers exist and how can they be modified to meet patient and provider needs? For example, if emergency room utilization is higher than necessary because people have difficulty calling their physicians, two processes might be changed: telephone triage and office hours.

B.   Structure/Prevention and Screening

Are there structural reasons that enrollees/members/patients do not receive the level of prevention and screening desirable for their age/sex cohorts? If so, what are the causes and how can they be addressed? For example, if a system's organizational structure includes an academic medical center and residents are responsible for prevention and screening, does the rotation schedule interfere with ongoing prevention and screening? If so, what administrative structure can be put in place to ensure that the desired goal is met?

C.   Structure/Disease Management

Has the system developed ways in which multidisciplinary teams of professionals can collaborate in providing care for people who already have or are at risk for medical problems such as asthma, chronic obstructive pulmonary disease, or cardiac problems? If not, what changes can it make?

K.   Process/Management of Enrollee Health

Do system policies for delivering care permit caregivers to take the time to work with enrollees to identify and meet health needs? For example, if a system has traditionally scheduled all visits with physicians and has been reluctant to use other professionals, it may want to reevaluate the policy and think about expanding staffing/scheduling to include non-physician providers such as nurse practitioners and physician assistants.

Process: *Process* applies to relationships between and among enrollees/patients, caregivers, administrative staff, and health plans. These relationships can affect outcomes, although some outcomes will occur regardless of process (Brook, McGlynn, and Cleary 1996). An example of process is access to care as measured by waiting time for appointments. If system administrative procedures and scheduling result in long waiting times that are unacceptable to enrollees, member retention is likely to be negatively affected.

Outcomes: The concept of *outcomes* in health care has many dimensions. Clinical outcomes apply to changes in the health status of individuals and/or populations. They can be determined by tracking clinical treatment and response to that treatment using generally accepted outcomes measures or quality indicators. Not all outcomes are clinical. There are financial outcomes as well—and much public criticism of the inappropriate precedence of financial over clinical outcomes.

Measurement Techniques   The measurement of structure, process, and outcomes will never be error free. Nonetheless, it can be valuable in helping clinicians and nonclinicians improve what they do and how they do it.

Brook, McGlynn, and Cleary (1996) suggest five basic questions to ask in assessing quality. If there are no prior standards or agreement on good or poor quality, three questions can be asked:

1.   Was the process of the delivery of care adequate?
2.   Could better care have improved the outcome?
3.   Given the process and outcome, was the overall quality of care satisfactory?

If a priori standards are in place, two kinds of questions might be asked:

1.   Did the process meet specific criteria agreed to in advance?
2.   Were the results of care not only consistent with criteria but also validated?

Using this basic framework, the measurement of quality depends on data. Potential sources of information are insurance company records used to reimburse claims, medical records maintained by caregivers, survey information, and direct observation of patients. A particularly difficult problem in integrated health care systems, especially those in their formative stages, is that information from different sources may not provide a clear picture of what happens to enrollees when they interact with different system components. Until their own information systems are able to assimilate raw data from multiple sources and integrate them, integrated health care systems may have difficulty understanding what really happens to the people for whose care they are responsible.

Reporting and Communication Integrated health care systems that understand the importance of quality devote attention to reporting and communication as well as to data collection. They gather and analyze information in ways that are responsive to user needs. For example, they may share information internally with both clinical and administrative staff to increase understanding of problem areas and achievements. They may also share information among system components so that each organization can understand the ways in which their relationships impact the process of providing patient care. Externally, quality information is shared with enrollees and with payers.

Development of Mechanisms for Quality Improvement

Of all of the challenges regarding quality that integrated health care systems must face, by far the most difficult is using information to make improvements on an ongoing basis. Information on quality is of little value unless it is purposefully applied. Some ways in which information on quality can be used to make improvements are credentialing, case management, clinical practice guidelines, and involvement of physicians in the broad spectrum of quality activities.

Credentialing Credentialing enables integrated health care systems to assess and monitor professional competence. Education, professional certification, and historical ability to operate within a specific budget are among the ways in which systems can evaluate potential providers.

Case Management Case management of both clinical and financial resources across the continuum of care is another way in which integrated health care systems can use information to manage patients.

Clinical Practice Guidelines   Clinical practice guidelines are systematically developed statements to assist practitioners' and enrollees' decisions about health care to be provided for specific clinical circumstances (Sundwall 1995). Because most guidelines focus on the processes of care, they are closely related to that aspect of quality management that focuses on process.

Physician Involvement   Physician involvement in and commitment to quality activities is by far the most important way for integrated health care systems to ensure ongoing attention to quality. Although, compared with other industries, health care is a newcomer to quality, important progress has been made in developing new techniques (Chassin 1996; Brook, McGlynn, and Cleary 1996). Furthermore, medicine has a long tradition of rigorous application of scientific methods to daily work. By virtue of training, experience, and professional relationships with patients, physicians are in a special position to apply their talent toward the improvement of patient care (Blumenthal and Epstein 1996).

FOCUS ON CREATING MARKET-DRIVEN VALUE

When organizations and individuals who are part of integrated health care systems are asked about their systems, most describe structure, governance, financing, and management. These topics are all necessary in systems formation, but they are internally focused on the organizations and individuals who are creating and operating the systems. They do not say much about "value" to the outside world that is positioned to buy or reject what systems have to offer. The real issue about value has been clearly framed by Donald Berwick: "Why should a 'customer' of an integrated health system care that we are doing this? How will this change and improve his or her experience?" (Berwick 1995).

Stated another way, if integrated systems want to earn long-term customer loyalty, they need to know what they are really selling. Customers do not need to know about system intricacies. Although customer priorities vary, all share a common need: They want products that suit their particular market niche, sold and delivered in a way that meets their needs, priced within their budgetary constraints—

all with minimal inconvenience (Coddington, Moore, and Fischer 1996).

Systems that view and manage themselves as integrated systems can do at least the following five things to promote value to customers; moreover, they are able to measure the results of what they do by looking at efficiency, satisfaction, clinical and process outcomes, and other results (Nolan and Berwick 1995):

- Facilitate scheduling by predicting demand for services. If systems offer a comprehensive array of services, they need to enable enrollees to make appointments for consultations, tests, and procedures without delay. A single appointment scheduling system, as well as ongoing adjustment of schedules to respond to predictable variations in demand, can help.
- Standardize processes linked to desired outcomes. The key word is "desired." Standardization for its own sake is not important; however, if it is linked to a desired clinical or administrative result, it should be done.
- Redesign the work flow so that the entire system, not just components, work smoothly.
- Focus on triaging enrollees to the appropriate setting for care, not on developing elaborate procedures for prior authorization.
- Treat customers as part of the system by designing processes and procedures to meet their needs.

Case 6-17 identifies systems that are attentive to market-driven value and that have developed specific indicators that help them retain internal and external accountability: Henry Ford Health System in Michigan, Dartmouth-Hitchcock Health System (Northern Region) in New England, and Mercy Health Services in Michigan (Shortell and others 1996).

References

American Hospital Association. 1993. *Transforming health care delivery: Toward community care networks*. Chicago: American Hospital Association.

Bennis, W, and B. Nanus. 1985. *Leaders: The strategies for taking charge*. New York: Harper & Row.

Berwick, D. M. 1995. How integration of care creates value. Presentation at Harvard Conference on Strategic Alliances, Boston, 1–3 November.

————. 1996. Quality of health care. Part 5: Payment by capitation and the quality of care. *New England Journal of Medicine* 335 (16): 1127–1231 (17 October).

Blumenthal, D. 1996a. Quality of health care. Part 1: Quality of care—what is it? *New England Journal of Medicine* 335 (12): 891–894 (14 September).

————. 1996b. Quality of health care. Part 4: The origins of the quality-of-care debate. *New England Journal of Medicine* 335 (15): 1146–1149 (10 October).

Blumenthal, D., and A. M. Epstein. 1996. Quality of health care. Part 6: The role of physicians in the future of quality management. *New England Journal of Medicine* 335 (17): 1328–1331 (24 October).

Brook, R. H., E. A. McGlynn, and P. D. Cleary. 1996. Quality of health care. Part 2: Measuring quality of care. *New England Journal of Medicine* 335 (13): 966–970 (26 September).

California purchasing co-op announces flat rates; unveils quality initiative. 1996. *BNAs Managed Care Reporter* 2 (32): 770–771 (7 August).

Chassin, M. R. 1996. Quality of health care. Part 3: Improving the quality of care. *New England Journal of Medicine* 335 (14): 1060–1063 (3 October).

Coddington, D. C., E. D. Moore, and E. A. Fischer. 1996. *Making integrated health care work.* Englewood, Colo.: Center for Research in Ambulatory Health Care Administration.

Cutler, C. M. 1995. What information do managers of health care organizations need to see? A physician manager's perspective. In *Measuring clinical care: A guide for physician executives,* edited by S. C. Schoenbaum. Tampa: American College of Physician Executives.

Darling, H. 1995. What information would purchasers like to see? In *Measuring clinical care: A guide for physician executives,* edited by S. C. Schoenbaum. Tampa: American College of Physician Executives.

Donabedian, A. 1982. *Explorations in quality assessment and monitoring.* 3 vols. Ann Arbor: Health Administration Press.

Fazen, M. 1994. *Managed care desk reference.* Dallas: HCS Publications.

Friendly Hills HealthCare Network. 1996. Duke University Medical Center site visit, 6May.

Gates, M. 1996. Information systems for integrated delivery systems. *Health System Leader* 3 (7): 4–12 (August–September).

Glaser, J. P. 1995. Strategic planning for information systems in integrated delivery systems. Presentation at Harvard Conference on Strategic Alliances, Boston, 1–3 November.

A glossary of information systems terms. 1996. *Health System Leader* 3 (7): 24–27 (August–September).

Greene, J. 1996. Power in the boardroom. *Modern Physician* 1 (1): 24 (October).

Halverson, P. K., G. P. Mays, A. D. Kaluzny, and T. B. Richards. 1997. Not-so-strange bedfellows: Models of interaction between managed care plans and public health agencies. *The Milbank Quarterly* 75 (1): 1–26.

Kemnitz, D. 1996. What employers are looking for. Presentation at 32nd Annual National Forum on Hospital and Health Affairs, 15 May, at Duke University, Durham, N.C.

Kongstvedt, P. R. 1993. *The managed health care handbook.* 2d ed. Gaithersburg, Md.: Aspen.

Kongstvedt, P. R., and R. Gates. 1996. Ten critical success factors for integrated delivery systems. Gaithersburg, Md.: Aspen.

Leider, H. L., and M. A. Bard. 1994. Leadership in managed care organizations: The role of the physician manager. In *The physician's guide to managed care,* edited by D. B. Nash. Gaithersburg, Md.: Aspen.

The Marshfield Clinic: Victory for integrated health care. 1995. *The Critical Edge.* Washington, D.C.: Coopers & Lybrand LLP and the Intergovernmental Health Policy Project.

McBride, S. 1996. Partnering for prevention. *PharmaCare Economics* 6 (5): S36–S39 (May).

Member complaints push HMOs to streamline referrals to specialists. 1996. *BNAs Managed Care Reporter* 2 (32): 758–760 (7 August).

Moore, J. D. 1996. Samaritan's revolution: New pay model aims to overhaul how workers think. *Modern Healthcare* 26 (31): 27–30 (29 July).

Mudd, S. C., ed. 1996. Creating healthier communities. *Healthcare Forum Journal* 39 (3): Special Report (May/June).

Nolan, T. W., and D. M. Berwick. 1995. Integration from the viewpoint of improvement. *Health System Leader* 2 (1): 14–19 (January/February).

Protecting patient confidentiality. 1996. *Healthcare Executive* 11 (2): 12–16 (March/April).

Reep, J. A. 1995. Who has the best information system for integrated health systems? Presentation at Integrated Healthcare Symposium, Aspen, Colo., 25–26 September.

Shortell, S. M., R. R. Gillies, D. C. Anderson, K. M. Erickson, and J. B. Mitchell. 1996. *Remaking health care in America: Building organized delivery systems.* San Francisco: Jossey-Bass.

Sundwall, D. N. 1995. Clinical guidelines: A tool for quality improvement. In *Measuring clinical care: A guide for physician executives,* edited by S. C. Schoenbaum. Tampa: American College of Physician Executives.

Van Etten, P. 1996. Spend more, get less. *Healthcare Forum Journal* 39 (6): 34–40 (November/December).

5

Barriers to Successful System Integration

INTRODUCTION

Although each integrated delivery system experiences unique growing pains, several barriers are common to all systems. These barriers may arise at a single point in time, or if left unaddressed, they may recur throughout the evolutionary process. This chapter describes common barriers and ways in which systems have addressed them. The discussion is organized according to the point in systems development at which they usually arise.

BARRIERS IN THE FORMATIVE STAGE

Barriers that often arise during a system's formative phase include failures to do the following:

■ Develop and communicate a vision of the end and interim states

- Identify the population(s) that the system expects to serve and outcomes that it wishes to achieve for each group
- Plan for capital needs
- Address differences in philosophy and culture
- Take the time to build trust
- Identify leadership skills and recruit/train talent to meet these needs

Failure to Develop and Communicate Vision of End and Interim States

A major obstacle for integrated health care systems, with and without the financing component, is failure to develop and communicate a long-term vision of their end and interim states. Like building a house without a design or a general contractor, this barrier can have major consequences. Lacking a strong foundation, the entire enterprise risks collapse.

Why the Barrier Exists   Integrated health care delivery systems fail to develop and communicate their long-term vision and interim stages for at least five reasons:

- Pressure of competition
- Tendency to reinvent the wheel
- Failure to distinguish transitional from long-term strategies
- Failure to distinguish between feasibility and planning
- Dependence on a visionary leader rather than a leadership team with vision

Pressure of competition: Most integrated health care systems form in response to actual or anticipated competition in the marketplace. In markets where multiple systems already compete, unaffiliated providers and insurers are often in a high state of anxiety. In less advanced markets, widely publicized expansion activities of large national health plans and of hospital and physician management companies puts fear in the hearts of regional and local providers. In an atmosphere of desperation, shotgun mergers and affiliations occur; suddenly there are "systems." In their haste, rather than planning their future, many of these new organizations simply act.

Tendency to reinvent the wheel: Although each integrated system is unique, the experiences of others can be helpful. Yet many systems pay little attention to what has gone before. "We are special," they say. "There's no need to ask anyone else." Even systems that are receptive about the experiences of others have difficulty obtaining information because competition discourages sharing the details that might help. Also, integrated health care systems are relatively new entities—in fact, many have taken shape within the past five years. Therefore very little information on their start-up and progress is available. Unfortunately, there are many case studies and not enough analysis.

Failure to distinguish transitional from long-term strategies: Another reason that integrated systems fail to plan their interim stages and end states is fixation on transitional strategies. Transitional strategies are not wrong. In fact, they are often necessary— provided their limitations are acknowledged.

The controversy over asset ownership versus virtual integration that is described in chapter I confuses many systems' thinking about their futures. Some systems believe that ownership and control are essential for success and that acquisitions will guarantee success. Other systems believe that relationships, not acquisition of assets, count more. But many systems do not deal with the question at all, thus remaining unsure as to whether their current course of action is a transitional or an end state.

PHOs are a good example. The 1995 Ernst & Young survey of PHOs suggests that these entities can help physicians and hospitals improve collaboration (Ernst & Young 1995). Yet many PHOs set overly ambitious goals of contracting with managed care plans and assuming financial risk, only to find that the market, financing sources, and regulators doubt PHOs' professional experience and financial stability. When PHOs do not achieve the goals they set for themselves, their participants must recognize that they are transitional strategies toward other end states.

Failure to distinguish between feasibility and planning: It would be interesting to take a poll of emerging integrated health care systems. An educated guess suggests that most have diligently commissioned feasibility studies to determine *if* they should form systems, but that many have not determined *how to* proceed once they are legally in place. As a result, many systems initiate multiple projects with no clear sense of how these efforts will unfold and relate to a larger purpose.

Dependence on a visionary leader rather than a leadership team with vision: Yet another reason why integrated systems do not distinguish between interim and end stages is leadership. Systems often form because a creative and visionary individual or a few key people take professional and personal risks to move the system. But a single individual or small cadre of visionaries cannot do it all. If the leadership lacks support from other capable team members who must manage operations and growth, the engine will have no train behind it.

Strategies for Clarifying and Communicating Vision   A number of methods can help systems ensure that they clarify interim and end states and that they communicate their direction both inside and outside the organization. Following are six suggestions:

- Build a participatory and ongoing long-range planning process into the system's development process
- Incorporate ongoing evaluation of system-building progress into the long-range planning process
- Engage outside consultants and advisors to guide the process of system development as well as to complete specific tasks
- Obtain information on other systems in a methodical and ongoing basis
- Develop, train, and coach a leadership team with vision
- Regularly communicate with external and internal audiences as the system grows

Build long-range planning into systems development: Long-range planning is the road map for building, operating, and expanding an integrated system. It is the tool with which each system can lay out its direction and monitor its progress as it develops. Planning must be part of the process, not an afterthought. It must be guided by competent senior leadership, and it must involve participation of representatives of many parts of the system. It must be dynamic, participatory, ongoing, and timely.

The strategic planning process at BJC in St. Louis exemplifies dynamic system planning (Tichacek 1997). Planning works at three levels. First, the board and CEO define mission, vision, and values. Second, a small executive council identifies critical success factors and key issues to be addressed. That group includes key physicians and other leaders. The third level of planning is done by the operating units, including six regions, service lines, and support functions. Over the years that BJC has formed and expanded, the planning process has changed to reflect the system's balance of centralization/decentralization. The system expects that planning will continue to evolve. Major factors that will affect the evolution are medical staff unification, alignment of physician incentives, better understanding of population-based care, and advances in information systems.

Incorporate evaluation of system-building progress into the planning process: As systems develop, they need to repeatedly ask themselves: "Are we moving toward a clear goal that we all support at the desired speed within budgetary constraints?" If the answer is no, the system must immediately reevaluate and take corrective action.

Two integrated systems that have measured their progress against long-range goals and made major midcourse corporate adjustments are Friendly Hills HealthCare Network in LaHabra, Calif., and Graduate Health System in Philadelphia. Friendly Hills first made and then severed an arrangement with an academic medical center that did not fit well with its long-range plans. It also tested several ownership arrangements. By 1996, it had an equity relationship with Caremark, now owned by MedPartners, Inc. During a decade-long process, Graduate Health System took numerous steps to grow and meet capital needs. Finally, in 1996, it turned the management of its operating units over to Allegheny Health, Education, and Research Foundation (Pallarito 1996).

Engage consultants and advisors to guide system development: External consultants and advisors can assist systems with the ongoing process of building a system, as well as with discrete legal, financial, and organizational tasks. Outsiders can contribute objectivity as well as experiences from other systems—two qualities that insiders are less likely to have.

However, the accountability of outside consultants and advisors must be seriously considered. If the consultant is engaged by an individual within the system who has a high personal stake in the system's planning process, the consultant's advice will be of less value to the system than if the consultant is accountable to a larger group charged with the responsibility for system planning. Sisters of Providence in Portland, Ore., used outside consultants to help it make major changes in its system. A case study published in 1994 (Kaluzny) provides details.

Obtain information on other systems: In a competitive market-place, insightful information on other systems will not be found in Web sites. Nevertheless, the information exists, and can be found by someone who is willing to search. Figure 5-1 lists recommended sources of this information.

The best way to learn about the experience of other integrated health care systems is to identify what information is needed and then pick up the telephone, old-fashioned though it may be. Colleagues at other systems are generally candid and helpful, provided their perceptions and insights remain confidential.

Develop leadership team with vision: Integrated health care systems must be built and managed. A visionary individual cannot make it happen; a leadership team with vision can. That team needs far more depth than the individuals who envision the future and close the deals on major acquisitions of system components. It needs people with operational experience, maturity, patience, and the ability to seek help when they do not know all the answers.

Sometimes existing personnel from within system components become effective members of the leadership team. When they do not, it is time to look outside for experienced individuals, not necessarily with health care backgrounds, who can do the job.

Regardless of which individuals assume particular responsibilities, skill building in teamwork can benefit the entire system. For example, one new integrated health care system recognized the importance of teamwork and identified the types of relationships it needed to address. Its long list included primary care/specialist caregivers, clinical administrative staff, members of the caregiver team (physician, unit nurse, clinical nurse specialist, social service, case manager, nutritionist), provider case manager/insurer case manager, clinicians/administrative staffs in different delivery sites, system and employee relationships, and system and community relationships.

Communicate regularly with external and internal audiences: After integrated systems engage in formal planning to outline their future, they can reinforce their plans with good communication inside and outside the organization. Common ways to do this include frequent retreats and presentations, regular newsletters, and regularly scheduled information sessions. For example, when Barnes-Jewish, Inc., and Christian Health Services merged to form

FIGURE 5-1.   Integrated Systems Information Sources

Books

Boland, P., ed. 1996. *The Capitation Sourcebook.* Berkeley, Calif.: Boland Healthcare, Inc.

Boland, P., ed. 1996. *Redesigning Healthcare Delivery.* Berkeley, Calif: Boland Healthcare, Inc.

Brown, M., ed. 1996. *Integrated Health Care Delivery: Theory, Practice, Evaluation, and Prognosis.* Gaithersburg, Md.: Aspen.

Coddington, D. C., K. D. Moore, and E. A. Fischer. 1996. *Making Integrated Health Care Work: Case Studies.* Englewood, Colo.: Center for Research in Ambulatory Health Care Administration.

Coddington, D. C., C. R. Chapman, and K. M. Pokowski. 1996. *Making Integrated Health Care Work: Case Studies.* Englewood, Colo.: Center for Research in Ambulatory Health Care Administration.

Conrad, D. A., and G. A. Hoare. 1994. *Strategic Alignment: Managing Integrated Health Systems.* Ann Arbor: AUPHA Press/Health Administration Press.

Goldstein, D. E. 1995. *Alliances: Strategies for Building Integrated Delivery Systems.* Gaithersburg, Md.: Aspen.

Kaluzny, A. D., H. S. Zuckerman, and T. C. Ricketts, eds. 1995. *Partners for the Dance: Forming Strategic Alliances in Health Care.* Ann Arbor: Health Administration Press.

Porter-O'Grady, T., and C. K. Wilson. 1995. *The Leadership Revolution in Health Care: Altering Systems, Changing Behaviors.* Gaithersburg, Md.: Aspen.

Senge, P. M. 1990. *The Fifth Discipline: The Art and Practice of The Learning Organization.* New York: Currency Doubleday.

Shortell, S. M., R. R. Gillies, D. A. Anderson, K. M. Erickson, and J. B. Mitchell. 1996. *Remaking Health Care in*

(Continued on next page)

FIGURE 5-1.   *(Continued)*

America: *Building Organized Delivery Systems.* San
Francisco: Jossey-Bass.

Newsletters and Periodicals

Health System Leader. Capitol Publications, Inc., 1101 King
St., Suite 444, Alexandria, Va. 22314; 800-655-5597.

Healthcare Forum Journal. 425 Market St., San Francisco,
Calif. 94105; 415-356-4470.

Hospital Integrated Care Report. Subscriptions Office, P.O.
Box 839, Lake Arrowhead, Calif. 92352.

Integrated Healthcare Report, P.O. Box 839, Lake
Arrowhead, Calif. 92352-0839; 909-336-1586.

Educational Programs

Integrated Healthcare Symposium. P.O. Box 839, Lake
Arrowhead, Calif. 92352.

New England Healthcare Assembly, P.O. Box 7100,
Portsmouth, N.H. 03802-7100; 603-422-6170.

The Health Care Forum, 425 Market St., 16th Floor, San
Francisco, Calif. 94105; 415-356-4300.

Selected Educational Organizations Conducting Integrated Health Care Systems Research

Arizona State University, School of Health Administration
and Policy, Tempe, Ariz.

Cecil G. Sheps Center for Health Services Research,
University of North Carolina at Chapel Hill, Chapel Hill,
N.C.: Arnold D. Kaluzny, PhD.

FIGURE 5·1. *(Continued)*

> J. L. Kellogg Graduate School of Management, Northwestern
> University, Evanston, Ill.: Stephen M. Shortell, PhD, and
> Robin R. Gillies, PhD.
>
> University of Pennsylvania, Wharton School, Leonard Davis
> Institute of Health Economics, Philadelphia: Lawton R.
> Burns, PhD.
>
> University of Washington, Department of Health Services/
> Washington Health Foundation, Seattle: Howard S.
> Zuckerman, PhD.

BJC Health System and later added the Missouri Baptist Health System and St. Louis Children's Hospital, the new organization developed a new communication plan. The four important messages were very different from the messages that each individual institution had previously emphasized: potential to reengineer health care delivery, define health care leadership, vision of the future, and partner in managing change (Martinson and Schall 1997).

Failure to Identify the Populations That a System Will Serve and the Desired Outcomes

News items about integrated health care systems generally highlight how many exist, how many are in the formative stages, and how many dollars these new entities represent. Relatively little is said about the ways in which integrated systems plan to impact the health and wellness of the enrollees for which they are formally responsible or of other populations. Failure to identify at an early stage the populations they will serve and the outcomes they wish to achieve presents a significant barrier for systems.

Why the Barrier Exists   Integrated health care systems underestimate the importance of population-based care for four reasons: historical delivery system orientation, balance between capitation and fee-for-service reimbursement, attitudes of private and public payers, and tension between marketing and management of care.

Historic delivery system orientation: Integrated health care systems that originate in the delivery system have historically provided care on demand to those people who had symptoms of illness and who sought care. If they have health prevention and wellness programs, these efforts may be slick marketing tools designed to retain current market share. The concept of identifying a population, assessing its health needs, and responding to those needs has probably not been a provider priority.

Traditional attitudes of public and private payers: Public and private payers have become increasingly distressed with their growing health care expenditures. Their response has been to pay less, shift risk, and clarify their expectations of quality and outcomes. Keeping populations healthy requires more than risk-shifting and report cards; it requires a positive commitment by payers that they value health and wellness. That commitment does not appear to be there—yet.

Impact of reimbursement methods: When integrated systems are reimbursed by capitation and other methods that transfer financial risk to them, they are more focused on keeping people healthy. However, in most situations, reimbursement is and will continue to be partially fee-for-service and partially risk-bearing, creating mixed financial incentives. In such transitional situations, providers do not commit themselves to assuming responsibility for health and wellness.

Tension between marketing and management of care: Integrated health care systems are not immune to the tension between growth and effective management that exists in every business. Sales and marketing efforts that produce enrollment growth generate revenue and allow systems to expand. Often, however, systems gain members well before they are internally prepared to assume responsibility for managing the health and wellness of enrollees. Systems' attention to the community at large, including but not limited to their own enrollees, is likely to come later.

Strategies for Initiating Population-Based Care

Integrated health care systems can initiate population-based care even before their information systems are in place. They can identify broad population groups and break those large groups into manageable cohorts. They can identify external expectations, learn from experienced health plans and systems, develop close working relationships with communities, incorporate health status assessments into system enrollment, and develop a basic plan for population-based care.

Identify broad population groups: Integrated health care systems can initiate population-based care for multiple groups. The top priority might be enrollees who officially belong to the system and for whom the system receives premium revenue. This group might be divided by age, sex, employee/dependent status, volume and cost of historical claims, disease categories, and chronic problems. The system can determine where it will focus and how it can tailor the organization of care to meet particular needs. Of secondary priority are groups for which a system might opt to provide care. Examples are the uninsured or underinsured.

Clarify external expectations: Systems that are sensitive to the market look hard at the external expectations for population-based care that are placed upon them directly or indirectly. Purchasers, purchasing groups, regulatory and licensing bodies, and other entities have become increasingly clear about their concerns and priorities, as described in chapter 2.

Learn from health plans and systems with experience: Selected managed care plans and integrated health care systems that have evolved over many years excel in population-based care. Systems that are new at this function should review what has already been accomplished and apply the knowledge to their own circumstances.

Develop close working relationships with communities: Population-based care provided by integrated health care systems has much in common with community efforts to identify health needs of specific populations and develop programs to address them. Systems should review the accomplishments of the "healthy communities" programs sponsored by both the American Hospital Association and the *Healthcare Forum Journal.* Especially when integrated systems enroll the Medicaid and Medicare populations, they should work closely with the public sector to jointly identify and meet needs. Case 6-14 and the section of case 6-2 on Carolinas HealthCare System describe ways in which several systems have linked population-based care with community health and advocacy.

Incorporate health status assessments into the enrollment process: An effective way for integrated health care systems to determine baseline health needs is to incorporate health status assessment into their enrollment processes. Effective assessment tools already exist; they can be used or modified depending on system goals. If enrollees make regular visits to physicians and other caregivers, assessments can be conducted or verified at the time of the visit. For the elderly, homebound, and those who do not make regular office visits, systems can send representatives to the home or institutional setting to perform the assessments.

Develop a basic plan: After an integrated system has completed health status assessments and evaluated the findings, it can begin to identify problems and prioritize interventions. The absence of complete information need not be an obstacle to laying out goals, tasks, time frame, and responsibilities.

Failure to Plan for Capital Needs

Failure to plan adequately for capital needs is a barrier that many systems first encounter during start-up. If the issue is not dealt with early enough, the problem is likely to continue throughout the system's evolution and impact its future course in an unanticipated and possibly negative way.

Why the Barrier Exists Two difficult issues obstruct integrated systems' planning for capital needs. First, if the concept of an integrated system is new to them, they may not know exactly what is required. Second, even if they are clear about what needs to be done, they may not know exactly what activities they will pursue.

Failure to identify needs for capital: Financial planning in general, including capital planning, cannot be done in a vacuum; it must be directly related to system planning. When an integrated health care system has no long-range plan or has a vague understanding of its future, preparation of a realistic capital plan is a challenging task.

Although a long-range plan can greatly facilitate capital planning, the plan may not identify operational costs. More up-front work may be necessary. For example, all systems need a strong primary care base. Systems that already include an existing well-balanced multipractice group will not need to spend capital dollars on practice acquisition. But most systems must incur a significant expense to build a physician base. A common mistake in capital budgeting is to estimate the dollars necessary for practice acquisition but to ignore other capital costs that will be incurred after the purchases have been made. Information systems, for example, must link acquired physicians with the rest of the system. The capital necessary to make these linkages is not always anticipated.

Failure to estimate the dollars needed: Once an integrated health care system has a reasonable idea of the tasks for which it needs capital, it must prepare realistic estimates of the dollars required. At this point, systems encounter two dilemmas. First, the individual or group of people responsible for systemwide capital planning may have little or no experience in such planning. Frequently, the capital planners have focused on capital needs for just one component of the system (often the hospital), but not the other components. Second, if the system is unfamiliar with the experiences of other systems, its capital planners will not be able to compare their projections with any kind of baseline information.

Strategies for Planning for Capital Needs   Integrated systems can take at least three steps to ensure that adequate capital planning begins during start-up and continues throughout the system's evolution. These are relating capital planning to long-range and operational planning, understanding sources of funding available to particular kinds of systems, and learning from the experience of others (Coddington, Moore, and Fischer 1996).

Relate capital planning to long-range and operational planning: Planning ahead for capital needs requires teamwork and frequent interaction between visionaries who see the end-state, planners who lay out the steps to get there, and operational and clinical personnel who understand what needs to be done. All these internal people, as well as outside consultants, must be involved in a system's capital planning process. If this internal synergy works well, a system can fine-tune its capital plan as it progresses.

Understand sources of capital: Identifying and estimating uses of capital is only half the challenge, however. An integrated system needs to understand available sources of capital and advantages and disadvantages of different options. If a system discovers that it has insufficient capital to survive and thrive, it may be necessary to develop partnership arrangements or change strategic direction to access sufficient funding.

Learn from others: Failure to anticipate capital needs has caused more than one system to founder, fail, or dramatically change course in midstream. Therefore, systems can benefit from the experiences of others as they do their capital planning. A productive way to gather information about capital planning in existing systems is to examine systems that have adequately anticipated their needs and those that have been less realistic.

Failure to Address Differences in Philosophy and Culture

Organizations differ in philosophy and culture. Philosophy applies to mission and goals. Culture applies to the values embodied in management style and the ways that people within the organization relate to one another and to the external world. Stated simply, culture is how things get done. Regardless of the method by which systems integrate, differences in philosophy and culture that remain unacknowledged and unaddressed can interfere with the substantive issues at hand.

Why the Barrier Exists   Many factors influence organizational philosophy and culture in all sectors of the economy. Among them are historical experience, management style, and reward systems. Two additional factors come into play in integrated health care: type of integration (for example, horizontal, vertical, functional, and so on), and sponsorship (such as for-profit/not-for-profit; religious/nonsectarian; or private/public).

Historic experience: Every organization has history. The circumstances of its origin and its tactics for growth, survival, and expansion impact employees' mindsets when the organization decides to integrate with other organizations. If the organization has experienced financial instability, integration may be perceived as salvation. But if the organization has been successful in achieving its mission and financial goals and there does not appear to be a crisis situation, coming together "for the greater good" may feel distasteful and confusing to employees at all levels. Individuals who have worked hard and met their organization's performance expectations are unsure where they will fit in the new scheme.

Management style: Although the CQI process, teamwork, and collaboration are repeatedly recommended as essential for systems success, not all organizations have adopted these approaches. In fact, many successful organizations have been led by smart, perceptive leaders whose top-down management styles have produced good results. When organizations accustomed to different management styles become involved in integrative activities, bewilderment, friction, and anger may surface. Two examples are academic medical centers and the Department of Veterans Affairs.

Academic medical centers have the potential to play a major role in the development of integrated health care systems, provided they can overcome the barriers to collaboration created by their historic management style. Particularly when academic medical centers embark on integration with for-profit companies, differences in management style become readily apparent. If left to fester, they impede progress. Specifically, academic medical centers place great value on consensus. They build it in meetings, hallway conversations, and less formal interactions. Traditionally, strong departmental chairs wield significant power; ceding some of their authority to others is difficult. Clarity in decision making and accountability are hard to find. By contrast, in a for-profit environment, hierarchy and decision making are very clear. If an academic medical center and a for-profit organization decide to work together, each may react negatively to the other's modus operandi before they jointly find a way to coexist and work toward common goals.

The Department of Veterans Affairs is currently working to integrate care through its regional Veterans Integrated Service Networks (VISNs). Historically, however, individual VA medical centers have enjoyed a great deal of autonomy. To achieve the goals set out for them, these individual organizations must embrace collaboration and consolidation with other VA facilities and learn from the experiences of the private sector.

Reward systems: Compensation systems reveal a great deal about organizational philosophy and culture. When integration occurs, differences in pay scales will surface. But pay scales are less important than reward systems. The type of reward, not the actual dollars, indicates what values are important. For example, some organizations have bonus systems that encourage outstanding behavior; others do not. Some organizations place financial value on teamwork; others do not. Sometimes, but not always, physician compensation recognizes quality factors such as access, patient satisfaction, and relationships with external utilization managers.

Type of integration: Integrated systems' abilities to identify and work through philosophical and cultural differences is directly affected by the type of integration that occurs. For example, if integration involves acquisition of assets and/or a former merger of different organizations, the new system often directs so much energy to the legal aspect of coming together that it neglects to deal with important basic differences. By contrast, in systems that are "virtually" integrated, relationships among the different parties are the focus from the outset. These systems are more likely to deal with philosophy and culture sooner rather than later.

Sponsorship: Finally, organizational sponsorship also impacts philosophy and culture. Systems with religious sponsorship bring with them a distinct approach to mission and ways of achieving it. Likewise, systems with physician sponsorship mirror physician styles of dealing with each other and with others.

Strategies for Addressing Differences in Philosophy and Culture   Although differences in philosophy and culture are less tangible than money, bricks, and mortar, they can be addressed methodically and successfully. One tool that can help systems create intra- and interorganizational cultural integration is the "core concepts" section of the Guidelines for the Malcolm Baldrige National Quality Award (see Fig. 5-2).

Other suggestions come from systems that have focused on culture and shared their strategies. These include early discussion of values, vision, and heritage; redesign of structures and systems to reflect new vision; creation of a sense of urgency for culture change; redesigning and merging clinical and operating systems; translation of values into measurable behaviors; attention to role models; creation of new incentives; and measurement of cultural shifts (Kennedy 1996).

FIGURE 5-2.   Guidelines for Malcolm Baldridge National
Quality Award: Core Concepts

Core Values and Concepts

Customer-driven quality
Leadership
Employee participation and development
Fast response
Design quality and prevention
Long range outlook
Management by fact
Partnership development
Corporate responsibility and citizenship

Criteria Framework

Senior excellence in leadership
Information and analysis
Strategic quality planning
Human resource development and management
Management of process quality
Quality and operational results
Customer focus and satisfaction

Source: National Institute of Standards and Technology. 1995. The Malcolm
Baldridge National Quality Award.

Failure to Take Time to Build Trust

Integrated systems that are asset-based and those that are virtually
integrated face a common barrier—the need to build trust. If they
do not take the time to build professional relationships among individuals in different components of the system, they will have difficulty working together to achieve common goals.

Unlike other barriers to the formation and maintenance of integrated health care systems, trust is a feeling that requires time to
cultivate and grow. No single activity performed by an individual
or group ensures trust. Trust requires attention at multiple levels.

When systems form, board members and senior management teams have frequent opportunities for personal interaction; they can begin to build relationships and trust. They can also set examples for the clinical, administrative, and support staff at all levels who will make integration work on a daily basis.

Failure to Identify Leadership Skills and Recruit/Train the Necessary Talent

Creation, operation, and expansion of integrated systems is complex. The stakes are high: many dollars, many people, and the potential to impact the health of individuals, populations, and communities. Although outstanding leadership is imperative, many systems fail to acknowledge the issue and address it methodically.

Why the Barrier Exists   Leadership problems in systems arise for many reasons, including lack of clear system direction, a common presumption that the system visionary will remain its leader, focus on individuals rather than on teamwork, and emphasis on structures and resources instead of skills.

Lack of clear system direction: Absence of clear vision and direction is directly related to leadership problems. When systems are not sure where they are headed, they cannot focus on the skills required to guide them toward their destination.

Presumption that the system visionary remains its leader: Integrated health care systems often begin because an individual with vision suggests a new approach. A common assumption is that that visionary will then move directly into the role of system chief executive officer and remain in that position. As described in chapter 3, however, the process by which integrated systems evolve is long and complex. Different leadership skills are required at different times.

When a system first forms, emphasis is on building internal and external relationships and on gaining sufficient market share to establish a break-even financial position. Skill in raising capital may also be important. When relationships, enrollment, and finances have stabilized, operational skills are needed. Still later, when internal operations are running smoothly, demonstration of quality becomes critical.

The same individual or senior management team may not have the skill set and flexibility to lead the integrated system through the entire developmental process.

Focus on individuals rather than teams: Competent leadership, important in all organizations, is not limited to a handful of senior individuals working in isolation. It involves individuals in key positions collaborating with one another as a team and setting a model for teamwork throughout the entire organization. Especially when they start, systems ignore the importance of teamwork. Restructuring, reengineering, and cost reduction generally consume a great deal of energy. Minimum attention is directed toward building the ultimate asset—the team that will ultimately make the difference.

Emphasis on structures and resources rather than skills: When systems are in their formative stages, large amounts of time, energy, and money are directed toward structures—that is, legal entities, governing boards, and management. Early efforts to eliminate duplication focus on resources. Yet after all is said and done, it is skills that count. Effective leaders understand the concept of a "learning organization" (Senge 1990). They make sure that employees at all levels of the organization learn new skills and continue their learning as the system evolves.

Strategies for Identifying Leadership Skills   Emerging integrated health care systems can deal constructively with leadership issues and obtain or develop the skills necessary to achieve their goals. Suggestions include conferring with other integrated health care systems, looking beyond the health care industry, contacting search firms that specialize in recruitment for integrated systems, inventorying skills and identifying gaps, and obtaining necessary skills by combining internal training and external recruitment.

Confer with other integrated health care systems: A good way to learn about the skills required to develop and manage integrated systems is to contact other systems. System leaders must talk with other current and former leaders about needs at different developmental stages. They must ask leaders in different professions how they develop and support their management teams. They must talk with human resources professionals and outside consultants about ways to teach and reward new skills and behaviors.

Look beyond the health care industry: Integration in the health care industry has much in common with consolidation in other sectors of the economy. Systems leaders must look to their colleagues in other industries for guidance and suggestions.

Contact search firms specializing in system recruitment: The speed with which integration in the health care industry is occurring has had major implications for health care professionals. Job stability and longevity are uncommon. As systems go through cycles of downsizing, reengineering, and gearing up, executive search firms are being called upon to assist with job definition as well as recruitment. Their experiences with different systems and with potential job candidates make them a good resource.

Identify necessary skills, current capabilities, and gaps between the two: Information from other integrated health care systems, from outside the health care industry, and from executive search firms can help systems determine what skills they need and how they might recruit and train staff. A starting point for discussion on senior leadership might be the following list of characteristics of effective leaders (Bennis and Nanus 1985):

- *Vision:* brings out the best in others; emphasizes emotional resources; expresses interest in others; demonstrates good judgment; expresses commitment to vision
- *Capability to provide meaning through communication:* problem-finder; interpreter; inspiration who pulls people forward
- *Trust through positioning:* capable of understanding the process to implement the vision
- *Deployment of self through positive self-regard:* good interpersonal leadership; contagious self-regard; willing to share uncertainties; accepting of failure as a learning tool; able to act as role model for a learning organization; capacity to be taught; long-range thinker who values innovation and creativity

Obtain necessary skills by combining recruitment and training: If a system is aware of the skills it needs, it can take two steps to obtain the talent. Outside recruitment is one option; many systems deliberately import experienced individuals and teams. Another strategy is internal training; some systems are committed to ongoing professional development of existing staff. Most systems combine outside recruitment with internal training.

BARRIERS DURING THE START-UP STAGE

After systems have legally formed, common barriers to progress include failures to do the following:

- Understand the importance of primary care
- Come to terms with governance
- Address inequities in resources, information, and benefits across system components

Failure to Understand the Importance of Primary Care

Primary care providers generally are the access points for enrollees. They may be formal "gatekeepers" who must authorize referrals to specialists, testing, hospitalization, and most other treatment. Even if they are not gatekeepers, they are the components of the integrated system with which most enrollees will have the most frequent interaction.

When systems are asked about their primary care provider strategy, they talk about building capacity, balancing the ratio of primary care to specialist physicians, placing primary care physicians in key governance and management positions, and compensating primary care physicians by reimbursement methods that recognize their role as managers and coordinators of care. Although these issues are important, there is more to it.

If primary care is to bring positive value to enrollees in integrated systems, primary care providers and specialists must develop a mutual understanding of each others' roles. For example, they may decide that enrollees with chronic and/or complex problems should have their care coordinated by specialist physicians. Enrollees as well as providers in different specialties must understand what primary care providers can and cannot do. Patient education can facilitate that learning process. Finally, components of the system other than the primary care providers themselves need to understand their pivotal role—and support it. System leaders must make sure that *everyone* understands the entire care delivery process.

Failure to Come to Terms with Governance Issues

When integrated health care systems establish themselves as legal entities, they often make early decisions about governance that create problems later. System leaders must constantly revisit governance issues to make sure that structure, processes, and board membership support the mission and goals. The importance of governance for long-term success cannot be overstated. "As integrated systems assume greater responsibility for the health status of a *defined* community, it will be governance that will carry much of the burden of transcending the needs and interests of both community and system" (Alexander, Zuckerman, and Pointer 1995).

Why the Barrier Exists   Integrated health care systems experience governance problems for many reasons. Common ones are failure to understand integration, board members' inexperience in the governance of complex organizations, lack of required skills and time commitments, difficulties with physicians involved in governance functions, and approaching governance as a short-term issue.

Failure to understand integration: When systems first form, different interest groups hear the message differently. As a result, when systems are in their early developmental stages, board members and management may have different perspectives about the system and their roles within it.

A common misperception by both governing boards and management is that integration automatically results from developing the *capacity* to deliver the continuum of care. Unless leaders pay close attention to system governance as well as to functional and clinical integration, the new system will be a system in name only and will not make an impact on the health of its enrollees and other populations.

Board members' inexperience in governance of complex organizations: Another common problem in system governance is board members' inexperience. For the sake of expedience and goodwill, the system board members may be former board members from system components. Those individuals understand board functions and responsibilities from an organization-specific, not a system-specific, perspective. Unless they have had other professional or personal experiences that have expanded their horizons, they will be most familiar with the governance of simple rather than complex organizations. Also, they will probably have minimal or no experience in making decisions about the structure, processes, and requirements for governance.

For example, representatives from physician group practices and other physician organizations are familiar with physician-only governance. They probably have had minimal experience in sharing governance responsibility with nonphysicians. Board members who come from not-for-profit community hospitals are likely to have had many years of experience in a single-purpose organization. They may have some familiarity with holding companies, but their geographic focus is probably narrow. As generous hospital supporters, they may have been called upon in the past to underwrite or sponsor unprofitable ventures, and they may not feel comfortable with a system that generates profits. System board members from nursing homes, home care agencies, and other small organizations may have been more intimately involved with day-to-day operational activities than are appropriate for a large system. Finally, if a system includes representatives from a health plan(s) as well as delivery system organization, those people will have had different governance experiences.

Lack of required skills and time commitments: Poor understanding of required board skills and time commitments also contributes to integrated systems' governance problems. As mentioned previously, systems often begin by placing board members from system components into system board slots. Systems leaders may later realize that governance could better serve the system if they more carefully examined required skills and time commitments and then selected qualified individuals.

Among the skills that systems have identified as important for board members are willingness to listen and learn, change, and take strategic and financial risks. With respect to time commitments, two issues are important. System board members must be prepared to invest time to listen and learn before they formally participate in decision making. Many systems attempt to reinforce systems thinking by asking board members to serve at multiple levels, rather than at a single level. This type of governance arrangement has many merits, but it also requires more time than many individuals can realistically give.

Difficulties with physicians in governance: Involvement of physicians in system governance is recognized as one of the more important strategies for integrating physicians into the fabric of an integrated system (Shortell and others 1996). Nonetheless, physician involvement generally brings problems that must be addressed. Overcoming physician fear and mistrust about working closely with nonphysicians, establishing appropriate and acceptable controls over the practice of medicine, encouraging physicians to engage in long-term rather than short-term thinking, and working through issues of physician selection for board participation are among the more prevalent concerns (Alexander, Zuckerman, and Pointer 1995).

Addressing governance as a short-term issue: Finally, systems often encounter governance problems if they put into place a particular structure, fill board slots, and breathe a sigh of relief because the job has been completed. Governance must support integrated systems as they change over time. It, too, must be subject to ongoing evaluation and modification.

Strategies for Addressing Governance Issues Integrated systems can take a number of steps to ensure that governance has a positive impact on the system. These include but are not limited to treating governance as an ongoing issue, clarifying and communicating the goals and issues in system governance, and building an educational component into the governance process.

Treat governance as an ongoing issue: Integrated systems are evolutionary entities. For governance to be appropriate at different stages of development, it, too, must change over time. Strategies that systems can take to ensure that governance is dynamic, not stagnant, include creation of a framework for ongoing discussion and evaluation of governance, identification of important governance issues, development of formal expectations for board members, use of an outside consultant or facilitator, imposition of term limits on board members, and creation of a full-time board chair and board staff.

Although the absence of effective strategic planning is a problem for many evolving integrated systems, those committed to formal planning can make the regular and automatic evaluation of governance an integral part of that process. If discussion and evaluation of governance starts early, it will be less offensive to individual board members whose personal expectations of tenure may ultimately be disappointed by changing organizational needs.

A second way in which systems can deal with governance on an ongoing basis is to anticipate and identify difficult issues as quickly as possible and communicate them throughout the system. For example, decisions about control, structure, board functioning, and board composition need to be made, reevaluated, and made again (Shortell and others 1996).

Third, systems can develop formal statements of expectations for board members. Periodic comparison of performance with expectations will strengthen their governance.

Fourth, in addition to engaging legal counsel to establish the entity, systems can engage outside consultants to assist with the ongoing process of governance evaluation. An outsider can bring knowledge about the experience of other systems to the table, and does not have the potential conflict of interest that a facilitator from within the system organization would have.

Fifth, systems can impose term limits for board members to make sure that as the system grows, it has the flexibility to select board members whose skills and experience best match its changing needs.

Finally, in recognition of the importance of governance, systems can fund a full-time board chairman and support staff.

Clarify and communicate goals and issues in system governance: The politics of board selection can be fierce. At times it overshadows intelligent discussion of the goals and issues of system governance. Examples of system governance goals are to facilitate those goals, formulate policy, provide a coherent framework for decision making, and provide oversight for the system. Important issues that warrant careful consideration include appropriate balance between centralized, regional, and local control, board size, and methods for addressing the balance between system goals and community needs.

Build education into governance: Education can have an impact on system governance. Regardless of their backgrounds prior to becoming a member of the systems board or one of its committees, all individuals involved in governance must have the opportunity to learn about the experiences of other systems. Within their own system, they must continuously learn new concepts so that they can maximize their effectiveness as individual board members and as part of the governance structure.

Failure to Address Inequities in Resources, Information, and Benefits

When different organizations come together to form an integrated health care system, three of the most difficult issues they will face are inequities in resources, information, and benefits. More often than not, however, these three topics are not addressed as quickly as they should be. Left as they are, they undermine other efforts.

Inequities in resources manifest themselves in several ways. The components of a system will vary in net worth and current operating position. Presumably they have come together to complement one another and to avoid unnecessary duplication. Nonetheless, the system component(s) with the most financial strength will be in a position to dominate the direction of the new organization. There will also be inequities in talent. Although every system component will have its chief executive officer and board, some will be stronger than others.

Information is a powerful tool. Some system components will have more and better integrated information and will have developed methods to use that information to their advantage. Those in a dominant position can hoard or share their data and their techniques for using it with others in the system who are less advanced.

Finally, system components will have different benefit structures. As suggested in chapter 4, not only salary structure but also reward systems will be different. Astute systems know that they must bring everyone onto a level playing field as quickly as possible.

BARRIERS DURING OPERATIONAL AND EXPANSION STAGES

Finally, systems will encounter obstacles during their expansion stages if they fail to do the following:

- Clarify lines of authority
- Orchestrate unique aspects of integrated systems: managing ongoing change, working with partners as opposed to subordinates, and managing internal and external relationships

Failure to Clarify Lines of Authority

The evolution of integrated health care systems occurs in incremental steps that take place over time. Time is an important factor of the growth process. During the evolutionary process, some relationships will appear to be clear. New organization charts, new titles, and new responsibilities will provide clues. Power and influence, however, will be less tangible. Lines of authority will become more clear as the new system determines its strategy and makes decisions.

Unclear authority in integrated systems has a domino effect that impacts people at many levels. Senior level managers who were accustomed to clarity about responsibilities and relationships and able to provide good direction to the people whom they supervised temporarily lose that clarity. They become unsure of their own roles and those of their colleagues and subordinates. Ambiguity of authority provokes tension, and people spend more energy worrying about the scope and limitations of their jobs than they spend on substantive issues. Productivity and creativity are placed on temporary hold.

When organizations change, unclear authority is inevitable; however, there are positive as well as negative ways to address that situation. The positive approach is to acknowledge it and allow board members, senior leaders, and other clinical, administrative, and support staff to express and work through their concerns. A negative way is to ignore it. The sidebar describes two integrated systems that took different approaches to the ambiguous authority issue.

Failure to Orchestrate the Unique Aspects of Integrated Systems

Managing an integrated health care system has many parallels with conducting an orchestra. Producing music that satisfies audience and musician expectations requires extraordinary sensitivity to internal skills and temperaments as well as external expectations.

■ **SIDEBAR**

Two Systems' Approaches to Unclear Lines of Authority

Integrated System A, like many systems throughout the country, believed in systems development by acquisition. It had sufficient capital to acquire primary care physician practices, invest in a health plan with which it formed a joint venture, and update support structures such as information systems. Employees in System A talked about the continuum of care, linkages across different sites, and the management of health and wellness. Full-page ads for System A appeared in the local, regional, and national media.

Internally, however, employees in System A struggled with ambiguous lines of authority. Although there were periodic reorganizations, there was no formal system governance or management. Separate components of the delivery system believed in their own self-importance and struggled to dominate the system. Lines of authority within components and across components were unclear. Elimination of positions through downsizing occurred on an ongoing basis, and fear of continued reduction in staffing pervaded the organization. There was little evidence of system planning and building a systems team. Authority, if and when one could find it, was ambiguous.

Integrated System B, located in the same market area as System A, took a different approach. System B believed in virtual integration. Its depth of health care services was dependent on relationships, not mergers and acquisitions. It developed strong partnerships with multiple managed care plans; none of those arrangements involved ownership. It had less capital than System A to spend on infrastructure. As a state-supported system, System B was committed to community health—long before the capitated method of reimbursement forced the issue.

Although employees of System B were not always certain where the organization was headed, they were not obsessed with power struggles and role ambiguity. The culture of the system was one of teamwork. Internal as well as external relationships were built on goodwill—"virtual integration." When responsibilities and roles changed, as they often did, System B talked openly about the difficulties involved.

Dealing with Ongoing Change Most health care professionals have years of experience working in relatively stable environments. Working in an integrated health care system requires the ability to function amidst ongoing change in the external environment and within the system itself.

The magnitude of change can be overwhelming. At Duke University Medical Center & Health System, six major changes in the following areas occurred within three years: (1) relationships between separate departments within the faculty practice plan; (2) relationships between the faculty practice plan and recently acquired community primary care physicians; (3) relationships between primary care and specialty providers; (4) relationships between the delivery system and 35,000 university employees who now had managed care insurance under a capitation arrangement; (5) relationships between the medical center and a joint venture insurance partner; and (6) the relationship between the physician and hospital components of the delivery system. These changes occurred simultaneously. Each change—and all of them together—required significant professional and personal adjustments (see chapter 7).

Working with Partners, Not Subordinates When integrated health care systems develop, individuals at many levels of the organization frequently struggle with a barrier that they have not previously encountered: sharing power among partners. At the senior executive level, individuals who are accustomed to supervising subordinates suddenly find themselves struggling with horizontal peer relationships. At the middle management level, managers who have spent their entire careers in discipline-specific activities suddenly realize that interdisciplinary teamwork is what counts to the new organization.

Bringing physicians into the equation is a challenge for many people. Developing cooperative relationships between providers, health plans, employers, and communities also creates difficulty for those who are unaccustomed to collaboration.

Systems leaders can deal with the partnership issue in several ways. They can make sure that the system's mission, goals, culture, values, governance, and management convey a partnership approach. They can also stretch beyond these formalities and concentrate on interpersonal relationships, the backbone of real partnership. The importance of collaboration among equals must permeate the entire system. The next sidebar describes a fictitious

■ **SIDEBAR**

System C: An Unwilling Collaborator

When System C first formed, its primary care capacity was inadequate to meet its enrollment goals. It therefore purchased the private practices of 50 physicians and organized them into a new entity, System C Primary Care Physicians, Inc. The new PCP entity reported to System C's flagship hospital, even though that institution had no prior experience in managing physician practices. The reporting relationship and the way in which hospital decisions were made created ill-will among the physicians. They were unable to convince hospital leaders to treat them as colleagues, not subordinates. Their expectations for active participation in their own governance were disappointed. Eventually the physicians notified Hospital C that they would join a competitor's system.

System C also had an insurance partner. Again, the flagship hospital in System C was not accustomed to sharing responsibility. Instead of looking for ways to collaborate with the health plan case/care managers, the hospital developed an elaborate list of requirements that the plan-based case managers would have to meet. The insurance partner had looked forward to procedures to facilitate staff interaction, not to barriers.

---

system that had difficulty developing partnership relationships with providers and with its insurance partner.

Managing Internal and External Relationships   A particularly challenging aspect of the management of integrated health care systems is the need to manage both internal and external relationships. Depending on the size and geographical scope of the system, the task can be formidable.

Internally, integrated systems must pay attention to multiple relationships, some of them within and across organizations. Externally, systems must manage relationships with a multitude of health plans and perhaps a health insurance partner. Relationships with governance and regulatory agencies, with agencies that look at quality, and with employers and/or employer coalitions are important. Finally, systems must take a careful look at community relationships and at enrollees' perceptions of the new entity.

One way that systems can manage internal relationships is to build organizational development into their process. With respect to external relationships, communication is key. Many people within a given system will have contacts in the external environment—but consistency is imperative.

References

Alexander, J. A., H. S. Zuckerman, and D. D. Pointer. 1995. The challenges of governing integrated health care systems. *Health Care Management Review* 20 (4): 68–81 (fall).

Bennis, W., and B. Nanus. 1985. *Leaders: The strategies for taking charge.* New York: Harper and Row.

Coddington, D. C., K. D. Moore, and E. A. Fischer. 1996. *Making integrated health care work.* Englewood, Colo.: Center for Research in Ambulatory Health Care Administration.

Ernst & Young LLP. 1995. *Physician-hospital organizations profile.* Washington, D.C.: Ernst & Young LLP.

Kaluzny, A. D. 1994. Centralization and decentralization in a vertically integrated system: The XYZ hospital corporation. In *Strategic alignment: Managing integrated health systems,* edited by D. A. Conrad and G. A. Hoare. Ann Arbor: AUPHA/Health Administration Press.

Kennedy, M. 1996. Creating a new postmerger culture. *Health System Leader* 3 (5): 4–11 (June).

Martinson, C. T., and T. Schall. 1997. Organizational landscaping 101: Planting the seeds with strategic communication. In *Anatomy of a merger: BJC Health System,* edited by W. M. Lerner. Chicago: Health Administration Press.

Pallarito, K. 1996. Allegheny adds to Philadelphia ranks. *Modern Healthcare* 26 (33): 10 (12 August).

Senge, P. M. 1990. *The fifth discipline: The art and practice of the learning organization.* New York: Currency Doubleday.

Shortell, S. M., R. R. Gillies, D. A. Anderson, K. M. Erickson, and J. B. Mitchell. 1996. *Remaking health care in America: Building organized delivery systems.* San Francisco: Jossey-Bass.

Tichacek, P. 1997. Strategic planning process. In *Anatomy of a merger: BJC Health System,* edited by W. M. Lerner. Chicago: Health Administration Press.

6

Cases Exemplifying Important Issues in Systems Integration

C hapter 6 includes 17 brief cases that illustrate many of the points made in chapters 1 through 5. Each case begins with a brief summary of the important issues. References for all cases appear at the end of the chapter.

Issue	Case	Health System(s)
Ongoing response to marketplace changes	6–1	Fallon
Alliances as a method of integration	6–2	Premier, Carolinas, Rehobeth McKinley
Functional integration	6–3	Baylor, Advocate
Market impact at different phases of system development	6–4	Duke, Vanderbilt, Boston metro area, Advocate, Allina, Sentara, Friendly Hills
Building primary care capacity	6–5	Lovelace, Duke, Partners
Combining not-for-profit and for-profit components	6–6	Tulane, Methodist

Issue	Case	Health System(s)
Combination versus separation of health care delivery and financing	6–7	Fallon, Mercy, Henry Ford, Duke, Graduate, Advocate
Competing systems that collaborate to improve community health	6–8	Council of Clinics, Health Partnership 2000, Oregon Health Systems in Collaboration
Philosophical commitment to integrated health care	6–9	Henry Ford
Changing culture	6–10	Henry Ford, Fairview
Clear purpose and vision	6–11	Baylor, Copley
Strong physician leadership	6–12	Henry Ford, Fairview, Friendly Hills, North Shore
Alignment of financial incentives and rewards for system performance	6–13	Samaritan
Focus on healthy communities	6–14	Group Health Cooperative, Laurel, Appalachian
Information systems and information technology	6–15	Advocate, Allina, Graduate
Commitment to quality	6–16	Lovelace, Presbyterian
Focus on market-driven value	6–17	Henry Ford, Dartmouth-Hitchcock, Mercy

CASE 6-1: ONGOING RESPONSE TO MARKETPLACE CHANGES

Well-established integrated health care systems repeatedly assess the market and reevaluate their strategy. This case describes the Fallon Healthcare System in Worcester, Mass., a system that combines health care delivery and financing.

The Fallon Healthcare System is a physician-directed integrated financing and delivery system. It evolved out of the Fallon Clinic and its HMO, the Fallon Community Health Plan. By summer 1996, the system included the clinic, the health plan, and the Saint Vincent Healthcare System, a corporate entity comprising Saint Vincent Hospital, three skilled nursing facilities, a home health care agency, a clinical laboratory, and other health care–related companies (the latter now owned by OrNda HealthCorp, since merged with Tenet Healthcare Corp.) (Plainte 1995; Southwick 1995). The system regards itself as "virtually integrated."

The Fallon Clinic, the backbone of the Fallon Healthcare System, is a multispecialty group practice with a long history. It was founded in 1929 as a surgical clinic in downtown Worcester. Subsequent reorganization of the group in 1970 and geographical expansion during the 1970s and 1980s led to the development of additional clinical sites and increases in staff. The merger of the clinic with Primary Care Physicians, a local group practice, strengthened the group's primary care capacity. By 1995, a total of 275 clinic physicians provided care at more than 30 locations. Another 1,500 physicians were affiliated with the system in an IPA.

After Fallon acquired the Saint Vincent Healthcare System, it sought a strategic partner to work with it. Exploratory talks with local and regional organizations did not produce the desired result—a partner that believed in the continuation of an integrated system, valued control by local physicians, and could provide the access to capital needed to actualize strategic plans. After a two-and-one-half-year search for the right match, Fallon selected OrNda HealthCorp, the third largest for-profit hospital management company in the country. (OrNda HealthCorp has since merged with Tenet Healthcare Corp.) Under an agreement approved by the state attorney general in August 1996, OrNda/Tenet now owns the Saint Vincent Healthcare System and a minority interest in the Fallon Clinic. Because the proposed deal involved conversion of a not-for-profit to a for-profit organization, issues regarding the provision of community benefits and local taxes had to be addressed (Podbielski 1996).

Unlike other health plans and health systems with which it competes for enrollment, the Fallon Healthcare System combines financing and delivery of care. The Fallon Community Health Plan was a thriving entity as the system developed, giving Fallon a head start in the marketplace. The health plan was established in 1977 through the efforts of the Fallon Clinic. It was the first HMO in central Massachusetts to provide direct enrollment and coverage to Medicaid and Medicare recipients in addition to small business and large group contracts. Over the years, the plan has grown in size; by 1995 enrollment was 175,000, including commercial and state employees as well as Medicaid and Medicare enrollees. The plan has added several options to expand the provider base, allowing members to choose a physician from the Fallon Clinic, the University of Massachusetts

Medical Center Faculty Practice, or an affiliated IPA physician. The plan has been recognized as one of the country's most effective health plans and has received national recognition for its quality assurance programs.

In fall 1999, the Fallon Healthcare System expects to open Medical City, a medical complex "designed for the 21st century," with a projected cost of more than $200 million. OrNda/Tenet will finance, construct, and manage the Medical City complex. Fallon Clinic's relationship with OrNda/Tenet will maximize its access to capital. The Commonwealth of Massachusetts and the city of Worcester shared in the cost of acquiring and preparing the Medical City site, and the project is expected to have a $1.6 billion spin-off in the Worcester County area over the next 10 years. When Medical City opens, more than 120 physicians, including 80 affiliated with the Fallon Clinic, will have offices at the new site. The clinic will continue to maintain primary care centers located in multiple locations. Saint Vincent Hospital will be downsized from 469 beds to 299 inpatient beds, of which 250 will be for acute care. Most important, the facility design will allow care to be patient-focused. Convenience for physicians and patients are important goals.

The plans for Medical City, however, will not guarantee desirable growth and continued success. The very structure and strategy that have resulted in success will need to be re-examined in the current market (Podbielski 1996). First, the Fallon Healthcare System includes both the financing and delivery of care. Its structure requires commitment to and dependence on a single health plan. Provider-based delivery systems that contract with many different health plans appear to be growing more quickly.

Second, the low price and high quality that once made Fallon a leader is not sufficient. By 1996, there was little or no premium differential among health plans and the quality of care did not appear to be a distinguishing factor for consumers. For the Fallon system, quality and value have translated into increasing enrollment. The system recently increased clinic and pharmacy hours and improved access to primary care physicians. The system also incorporated incentives related to enrollee satisfaction into its compensation plan for all employees.

Third, with respect to the Medicare risk product, the Fallon physician network is quite large, but other risk products offered by HMO Blue, Harvard Pilgrim Health Care, and Tufts Associated Health Plan offer an even greater choice of physicians. Fallon continues to rethink both its strategy for the commercial and senior markets and ways to enhance its products to continue to increase market share.

CASE 6-2: ALLIANCES AS A METHOD OF INTEGRATION

Alliances can be an effective way for components of a system to come together. They depend on relationships and enable members to pool resources, jointly explore opportunities, and link activities through partnership arrangements. They permit pursuit of activities that might not be done alone. They also offer opportunities for mutual learning (Kanter and Stein 1993). This case describes three alliances: Premier, headquartered in North Carolina; Carolinas HealthCare System in North Carolina; and Rehobeth McKinley Christian Health Care Services in New Mexico (an alliance that has resulted in a merger).

Premier

Premier is the country's largest alliance. As of January 1997, it represented more than 240 owner systems that in turn owned or operated 700 institutions. Premier also has affiliations with another 1,100 hospitals. Membership is diverse, including multihospital systems serving entire regions, academic medical centers, urban acute care facilities, and rural community hospitals. These members operate hospitals, health plans, skilled nursing facilities, rehabilitation facilities, home health agencies, and physician practices.

The alliance offers members leverage, opportunities for cost reduction, strategies for delivery system development and integration, technology management, decision support tools, and many opportunities for networking and knowledge transfer. All these services can assist members in achieving health status improvement and cost reduction goals (Yandell 1997).

The alliance is only 18 months old. It was created in January 1996 through a merger of Premier Health Alliance, American Healthcare Systems, and SunHealth Alliance. Each of the three alliances had already achieved success within different geographical regions of the country when they decided to come together. Although skeptics have expressed doubt about the ability of such a large alliance to continue to meet member needs, first-year results have been impressive. Although some organizations that were formerly members of the three separate alliances have resigned from the new Premier, total membership has increased slightly. The group purchasing program, one of Premier's major attractions, exceeded original estimates by 30 percent and saved a total of $650 million. The takeover of purchasing for the Greater New York Hospital Association was a major accomplishment, as were a seven-year $7.2 billion deal with Baxter International-Allegiance and a five-year agreement with Johnson & Johnson (Stodghill 1996). Figures 6-1, 6-2, and 6-3 include details on foundation statement/core ideology, alliance overview, and first-year corporate accomplishments (Yandell 1997).

Group purchasing is one of many Premier services; expansion plans call for continued development of a physician practice management unit, formation of a limited liability corporation to handle capital equipment planning and purchasing, addition of new board members with Wall Street connections, and support of a research firm (Hensley 1997a, 1997b).

With respect to physician practice management (PPM), Premier expects to compete with the country's largest companies. One of the hurdles it must overcome is physician skepticism about practice management by a hospital—or by an alliance with hospital ownership. The alliance plans to give physicians, hospitals, and Premier equal stakes in a regional PPM; equity stakes will not allow domination by one of the partners. Over the long term, the regional PPMs will be combined into a national company and floated as a publicly traded stock corporation, hopefully within six years.

Premier Technology Management is the new limited liability corporation that combines technology assessment, capital equipment purchasing, and biomedical service and maintenance insurance. The goal is to help members better manage the capital equipment life cycle. As part of a pilot project, 50 alliance members are supplying their capital budget forecasts to Premier so that purchase planning can be done across the alliance.

Carolinas HealthCare System

Carolinas HealthCare System (CHS), formerly the Charlotte-Mecklenburg Hospital Authority, is a quasi-governmental integrated regional health care system providing care to residents of

FIGURE 6-1.   Premier Foundation Statement: Core Ideology

Core Values

Integrity of the individual and the enterprise
Enduring respect for others' worth and rights and for the
principles that uphold our communities
A passion for performance and a bias for action: creating real
value, engaging change, leading the pace

Core Purpose

To improve the health of communities

Core Roles of the Enterprise

Producing quality improvements and cost savings across the
continuum of health care
Facilitating the rapid transfer of knowledge and experience
Providing vehicles for collective strategies
Providing alternate revenue sources

Source: Premier Public Relations Material, 1997.

12 counties in North and South Carolina. Although it is not a formal alliance, it brings together both private and public sectors, urban and rural providers, and direct and indirect purchasers of care in arrangements made many years before the community-focused integrated health care systems developing today.

From the perspective of the president and CEO of CHS, keys to the system's longevity and accomplishments include the following (Nurkin 1995):

- Corporate governance and attitudes that are conducive to nontraditional approaches to policy making
- Flexible and nontraditional approaches to management of diverse, sometimes conflicting, efforts and people
- Financial stability of the coordinating entity

FIGURE 6-2. Premier Overview

Leverage

Group purchasing at levels that enable members to achieve
tremendous economic rewards
Intellectual capital founded in the knowledge of the alliance's
leaders, hospital employees, and staff
Comparative data and benchmarking expertise that give
members a competitive advantage
Market presence that allows Premier owners and affiliates to
reach out to U.S. business and influence its health care
provider choices
A Washington office that maintains an active advocacy program
designed to influence legislative and regulatory outcomes

Cost Reduction: Use Tools Available through Premier to Realize the Following Benefits

Reduce expenses by comparing services and labor costs
among similar institutions.
Achieve some of the industry's lowest pricing through the group
purchase of medical/surgical supplies, pharmaceuticals,
lab, and dietary products.
Streamline clinical and operational processes through
reengineering techniques, benchmarking, and other
performance improvement services.
Reduce equipment purchase, repair, and maintenance
expenses through technology assessment services and
medical equipment maintenance programs.
Lower insurance premiums by purchasing coverage in
conjunction with other alliance organizations.

System Development and Integration

Prepare for the next step in managed care.
Plan and implement information systems that can support
sophisticated transfer of data among and outside system sites.

FIGURE 6-2. *(Continued)*

Offer practice management services to local physicians.
Learn how to integrate clinical and business processes across
the continuum of care.

Technology Management

Research resources to assess new and emerging equipment
technologies and clinical procedures.
Maintain and repair biomedical and imaging equipment to
ensure the safety of patients and employees.
Access competitive medical equipment parts distributorship 24
hours a day.
Provide cost-effective options for clinical engineering
department management and equipment maintenance
agreements.

Knowledge Transfer

Access or participate in clinical and operational benchmarking
studies.
Attend peer group meetings and educational conferences for
administration, department managers, physicians, and
nurse executives.
Utilize library resources, including custom research, books,
reports, tapes, and periodicals.
Attend government conferences and shareholder meetings to
network with colleagues.
Directly interact with Premier through regional executives and
materials services liaisons.

Source: Premier Public Relations Material, 1997.

- Patience
- Tolerance for ambiguity

CHS was established in 1949 under the North Carolina Hospital
Authority Act. Technically, it is a unit of state government operating

FIGURE 6-3. First-Year Progress at Premier

January 1996	April 1997
Characterized by size and uncertainty	Solidification of management team, unification of business plan and budget, and development of new, enhanced, and core heritage activities
Not well known outside health care	Living up to name with well-established name and logo: Positive articles published in national magazines and newspapers; national politicians have recognized importance; and interest at key owner, business partner, and federation meetings demonstrated by record attendance
Lacking new materials contracts	Improved materials contracts, including those with Baxter and other companies, have saved owners millions of dollars
Maintaining three separate payroll systems	Single uniform system permits continued receipt of uninterrupted service from accounting and human resources
Lacking consistent titles, compensation, and retirement plan benefits	Three-year transition plan being implemented to make titles, compensation, and benefits consistent
Lacking defined corporate policies and procedures	Policy manual establishes corporate procedures
Using different telephone equipment, voice mail, software, computer hardware, and E-mail	Single telephone and voice mail system; more uniform software standards; a wide-area network; and video teleconferencing
Operating with different standards for office furniture and not using planning to expand office space to address existing corporate space well	Using standard office fixture standards that enable future growth

Source: Yandell, L. 1997. Interview by author. Premier, Charlotte, N.C., 9 April.

as a not-for-profit corporation (Keener, Baker, and Mays 1997). The authority began with Charlotte Memorial Hospital, now called Carolinas Medical Center. Today CHS includes that tertiary care hospital, regional hospitals, long-term care facilities, a home health agency, and a network of more than 400 physicians. CHS has an annual budget of $1.2 billion and 9,000 employees.

The relationship between CHS and components of the system are varied. CHS owns, leases, manages, or has joint ventures with 12 hospitals. It is discussing an alliance with three other academic medical centers. With respect to managed care, the system has agreements with various managed health care plans and contracts directly with several large employers. It holds an ownership share in one health plan and is entering into a joint venture with another. The physicians owned by the system are mostly but not exclusively primary care practitioners. Many of those physicians are part of the Davidson Clinic or Charlotte Medical Clinic (White 1997).

The public-private partnership arrangement that CHS has with Mecklenburg County has evolved over time. In many respects, it is a model for collaboration in other communities. During a 15-year period, the county had privatized health services such as a rest home, a nursing home, and a mental health center. CHS's largest hospital had provided medical control for the area emergency medical system, served as a site for county social workers to enroll hospital patients in Medicaid managed care, and provided care to jail inmates. In 1995, CHS and the county signed a five-year interlocal contractual arrangement extending from 1995 to 2001. The county pays CHS a fixed fee to provide specific public health services traditionally offered by the county health department. The services provided by CHS represent 80 percent of the health department's staff and resources and include direct clinical services, community services, support services, and public health assessment and policy development activities. The contracted services are housed within the CHS department of public health, Division of Education. Health department staff were given the opportunity to work for CHS. The county health department retains primary responsibility for managing and overseeing the CHS contract and for providing those services that legally could not be contracted out to CHS (Keener, Baker, and Mays 1997).

The CHS/Mecklenburg County contractual arrangement includes an interesting financial provision that enables it to function much like capitation. For the entire term of the contract, county funding for all contracted services is fixed at the 1995–1996 fiscal year level. Thus, CHS has a financial incentive to improve the efficiency with which care is provided.

Quality should be important in all integrated health care systems. Particularly in an initiative that involves both public and private sectors, it is imperative to balance public health goals with objectives regarding efficient and cost-effective delivery of care. CHS and Mecklenburg County approach quality from three directions. The county governance and advisory structure is the basic system for quality management. An internal monitoring system is jointly maintained by a university-based health service research center and the system's own research institute. Finally, the state health agency has developed a local public health care report (Keener, Baker, and Mays 1997).

Urban-rural relationships in CHS as well as the public-private aspect are interesting. A federal grant enabled the hospital authority to plan an alliance between rural and urban hospitals. Today rural members of the system participate in the determination of programs and strategies that are appropriate for their facilities.

Rehobeth McKinley Christian Health Care Services: Alliance as a Prelude to Merger

The alliance concept is by no means limited to large systems or to urban areas. An example of a rural "alliance" that eventually led to merger is Rehobeth McKinley Christian Health Care Services (RMCHCS) in west central New Mexico (American Hospital Association 1993).

The geographic setting for the RMCHCS is McKinley County, N.M., an area adjacent to both the Navajo Reservation and the Zuni Pueblo. The total population of the county is 62,000, of whom approximately 20,000 live in Gallup. Although the 200,000 Navahos and 7,000–8,000 Zunis do qualify for care at the Indian Health Services Hospital, that institution does not provide a full spectrum of care. As a result, many Native Americans seek some of their care at other facilities.

A major health issue for the community is alcoholism; McKinley County has one of the worst problems in the country. The magnitude of the problem and the county's historic inability to improve the situation has created a drain on both health and other community resources.

Historically, two nonfederal hospitals served both non–Native American and Native American populations. Rehobeth Christian Hospital had 41 beds; county-owned McKinley General Hospital in Gallup had 71 beds. Rehobeth Christian had ties to the Board of Home Missions of the Christian Reformed Church. A group of physicians, known as the Luke Society, provided care on a volunteer basis. McKinley General, located seven miles from Rehobeth Christian, had originally been a Catholic hospital, but management responsibility had been assumed by Southwest Community Health Services in Albuquerque.

In the mid-1970s, both institutions experienced financial difficulties. Although they served the same population, cooperation was threatened by major barriers. One problem was differences of opinion on the importance of religion. Rehobeth Christian feared dilution of the missionary zeal so important to it. Also, members of the Rehobeth community who had contributed financially to the erection of a new building did not want to see the facility's values compromised. McKinley General supporters feared imposition of Christian missionary ideals on hospital operations. Nonetheless, visionaries within both organizations continued to encourage collaboration.

The first step for the two hospitals was to create the Area Health Cooperation Committee, their alliance. The committee's goal was to formulate cooperative activities to better use the resources of both institutions. Although the committee found several cooperative projects, ultimately it engaged an outside consultant. His advice was to talk seriously about merger or risk disintegration of the basic services of both hospitals.

Despite major obstacles, merger discussions proceeded. "Divine providence," focus on similarities rather than differences, exclusion of local government representatives from negotiations, limitation of physician representatives to the two chiefs of staff, and development of a small working group were factors that facilitated progress. The small working group sought input from outsiders, and communicated openly.

The process by which the two hospitals moved toward merger was slow and rocky; it took four years. There were several false starts when boards of each institution changed their minds. Eventually, a new administrator was recruited. However, when he arrived, he found that the two existing boards had created a new board but not yet dissolved themselves!

Although the difficulties encountered during the alliance phase did not bode well for the merger, fears were never realized. Board members of the new entity were supportive of the decision to merge and dealt with negativism. Their decision to consolidate services was implemented without any service discontinuation. A particularly difficult aspect was related to the merger of the medical staffs. There had been a joint commitment that no one would lose jobs as a result of the merger. Although maintaining that position was difficult, by the end of the first year, only 20 people had lost their jobs.

After a year of reorganization and consolidation, RMCHCS turned to service enhancement. Highlights of its initial efforts included a women's health service, home health service (including transportation), improved access to renal dialysis and CAT scan, cooperation with a private not-for-profit clinic, and major improvements in the provision of serves to treat alcoholism. Within three years, the new entity had achieved financial stability.

CASE 6-3: FUNCTIONAL INTEGRATION

In the longitudinal study of integrated health care systems conducted by Stephen Shortell and his colleagues, the team identified systems that demonstrated significant progress with functional integration (Shortell and others 1996). Two of these were Baylor Health Care System in Texas and Advocate Health Care in Illinois.

Baylor Health Care System

Baylor in Dallas has often been regarded as a model of integration for both academic and nonacademic medical centers. When the organization decided to build an integrated delivery system, it faced four major hurdles. First, the market was not yet at the point in growth of managed care to demand change, and exerted minimal pressure to contain the cost of health care. Second, Baylor's excellent clinical reputation made it difficult internally to motivate change. Third, Baylor University Medical Center dominated the system. Fourth, the organization lacked a consistent strategic vision.

To launch the integration effort correctly, Baylor's leaders devoted significant time and energy to system strategic planning, a cornerstone of functional integration. They created a high-level System Integration Action Team, including 28 employees and physicians directed by the system senior executive vice president and chief operating officer. The group met for 18 months to focus on where the system as a whole would go and how it would get there. The group developed the following seven core system processes:

- Managing illness
- Optimizing health and wellness
- Coordinating member education and access to care
- Developing, updating, and communicating system strategies
- Capturing the market
- Assessing and managing risk
- Managing resources to support the core processes

Advocate Health Care

Advocate Health Care in Park Ridge, Ill., is the product of a 1995 merger between Evangelical Health System (EHS) and Lutheran General Health system (LGHS). Functional integration was addressed prior to merger and has continued.

Before the merger, EHS looked carefully at the way in which its separate operating components functioned as a system and identified opportunities for improvement. These included development of a system culture, clear communication of the goals and processes of integration, introduction of financial incentives based on system performance, and use of programs on diversity in the workplace. The CQI/TQM process was an important part of the effort. Using CQI/TQM methods, EHS developed training programs on system mission, values, and standards. These programs were targeted at all levels of employees and permitted people in different operational units to participate in shared learning experiences. Eventually, these educational programs were formalized into EHS University, enabling employees to earn continuing education unit credits. At a senior level, financial incentives were related to systemwide performance.

Since the merger of EHS and LGHS, Advocate has continued to focus on functional integration, addressing conceptual, economic, and cultural factors. To some extent it has had to go backward before it moves forward. Features of the Advocate approach to functional integration are regional management teams located at corporate headquarters, programs directed toward development of physician executives, asset merger and consolidation of financials, creation of a single board, and creation of a "super" PHO to which local PHOs relate.

CASE 6-4: MARKET IMPACT AT DIFFERENT PHASES OF SYSTEM DEVELOPMENT

Market forces impact integrated systems throughout their evolution. This case describes market influence on systems at different developmental stages. Examples of market impact on system initiation can be seen in Duke University Medical Center & Health System in North Carolina; Vanderbilt University Hospital and Clinic in Tennessee; and the Boston metropolitan area. Advocate Health Care in Illinois, Allina Health System in Minnesota, and Sentara Health System in Virginia are good examples of market influence at midcourse in systems development. Market influence in mature markets can be seen in Friendly Hills HealthCare Network in California.

Market Incentive to Initiate Systems Development

Duke University Medical Center & Health System In 1992, Duke University Medical Center (DUMC) in Durham, N.C., embarked on a strategy to build an integrated health care delivery system. At the time, DUMC was financially sound and enjoyed an outstanding reputation as a tertiary referral center. Managed care was in its infancy in North Carolina. Although a number of commercial health plans described themselves as "managed care" plans, most were PPOs. In the public sector, the "managed" Medicaid plan, like the commercial plans, lacked most of the features associated with strong managed care. A small number of Medicare recipients participated in risk programs.

Given the external market, there was minimal internal emphasis on cost control/reduction and quality of care to meet payer and consumer standards. When DUMC looked outside itself and speculated on future market changes, it realized that the high cost of teaching and its historic emphasis on specialty rather than primary care would not take it successfully into the future. These market factors stimulated the strengthening of primary care and the building of the Duke University Medical Center & Health System (Rogers, Snyderman, and Rogers 1994), which is the focus of chapter 7.

Vanderbilt University Hospital and Clinic   Retooling any academic health center/system is a complex challenge. Vanderbilt University Hospital and Clinic in Nashville, Tenn., has undergone extensive retooling of its delivery of care in a process that began in 1989 and has continued to respond to market forces (Baker and Dubree 1996). When the process began, managed care was not particularly important in the market, but the organization was nonetheless concerned about negative perceptions of the delivery of patient care by both patients and staff. Within seven years, managed care had become very important in Tennessee, and Vanderbilt was well positioned because of its earlier attention to changing market forces.

For Vanderbilt and many other academic medical centers/ health systems, the impetus to change is often realized through grant money and pilot programs rather than a conscious organizational commitment to change. Supported by the Robert Wood Johnson Foundation and Pew Charitable Trust, Vanderbilt began its efforts to improve patient care and the quality of work life by establishing a Center for Patient Care Innovation.

Initially Vanderbilt planned to focus on nursing; however, it soon became clear that other disciplines and departments needed to be involved. At first, the Center for Patient Care Innovation provided assistance to internal teams to improve operations in a cost-neutral way. But the governor's introduction of TennCare Medicaid managed care in 1993 made cost reduction, not cost neutrality, an imperative.

Vanderbilt's pilot for redesigning care was the Orthopedic Redesign Project. That project showed that work redesign could increase quality, decrease cost, and improve patient, staff, and physician satisfaction. Positive results from the project led to a larger operations improvement effort in both hospital and clinic.

Vanderbilt then turned its attention to restructuring. Inpatient care was the focus, and new patient care delivery models in 26 units and six central departments were built. Other important components of Vanderbilt's reorganization of care were the following:

- Collaborative care: agreed-upon process to provide care to different groups/types of patients
- Case management: coordination of care during an entire episode of illness by designated care managers to optimize clinical and financial patient outcomes

However, even those efforts were not sufficient to respond to the market. The locus of care was moving from inpatient to outpatient care; Vanderbilt's Collaborative Organizational Design acknowledged that shift. The next challenges would be changes in physician practice, and new physician work groups were set up to parallel those at the hospital.

Boston Metropolitan Area   A third example of market impact on systems formation is Boston. In the early 1990s, both the public and private sectors underwent major changes in health insurance. The Commonwealth of Massachusetts had demonstrated its savvy as a purchaser of health insurance for public employees. It then developed and implemented a mandatory statewide managed Medicaid program. Shortly thereafter, the second largest HMO in the state, Bay State Health Care, was purchased by Blue Cross and Blue Shield of Massachusetts. Those events resulted in a sudden and almost simultaneous reduction in provider reimbursement. Many providers who cared for large numbers of Medicaid clients and Bay State enrollees experienced an unexpected large decrease in reimbursement.

These events made providers certain that the influence of large health plans would continue to grow unless they took the initiative to develop provider-dominated regional systems. Within a few years, three strong provider-based regional systems emerged: Partners HealthCare System, Inc.; CareGroup Health Network, Inc. (formerly Pathway); and Lahey-Hitchcock Clinic System. Strong health plans included Harvard Pilgrim Health Plan, Tufts Associated Health Plan, and the Fallon Health Plan (part of the Fallon Healthcare System). Blue Cross and Blue Shield of Massachusetts began moving toward regional collaboration with other New England Blue Cross plans.

Market Influence at Midcourse in Systems Development

Advocate Health Care   The external market also impacts integrated systems after the point at which they form. In the

Chicago area, both Lutheran General Health System and Evangelical Health System were successful systems prior to their 1995 merger into Advocate Health Care. Both systems believed they needed greater market share to thrive; hence their decision to combine into a new larger entity. The merger enabled Advocate to offer care in a 60-mile area in north, south, and central Chicago.

Allina Health System   Allina Health System in Minnesota was created by merging HealthSpan Hospital System and the Medica Health Plan. Both had been successful, but neither felt secure enough in the marketplace to remain as it was. In anticipation of many market advantages, the merger partners addressed the following questions (Rainmakers 1995):

- Could the new entity improve community health in a heterogeneous geographical area that included very poor and underserved communities?
- Could a large $2 billion organization respond to payers' and consumers' needs?
- Would such a large system become impersonal in its response to the market?

Sentara Health System   Sentara Health System in Norfolk, Va., includes four owned hospitals, one joint-venture hospital, 140 employed physicians, and six insurance products with a total enrollment of 228,000. The system provides care to more than 2 million people in Virginia and North Carolina. (In spring 1997, Sentara and Tidewater Health Care announced a proposed merger.)

In 1995, Sentara was in sound financial shape, but its leadership believed that its decentralized structure required modification. The system embarked on a five-year repositioning program known internally as "Reinventing Sentara" (Scott 1997). The goal is to integrate both services and facilities, and the strategy for making the changes relies heavily upon operational people. The four areas of focus are governance, physician involvement, cost reduction, and growth of managed care enrollment and capitation arrangements.

Governance: Six subsidiary boards and a holding company have been consolidated into a single system board. The number of standing committees has been reduced and an executive council has been created.

Physician involvement: The new executive council consists of four system executives and four physicians, thus giving physicians input into governance and management, as well as equal partnership. Physicians have assumed different leadership roles. For example, one is responsible for physician education; another works with the system's chief information officer on clinical information systems.

Cost reduction: Four full-time reengineering teams of managers willing to give up their previous positions were designated to identify processes that could be improved, develop a plan, and work with other operational staff to implement changes. Among the major projects were hospital, laboratory, and pharmacy consolidation. The team approach was so successful that it will become a permanent feature of the system. New managers will replace outgoing members of the reengineering teams and, like their predecessors, will serve from 18 to 24 months.

Growth of managed care enrollment: Sentara's strategy to compete with other systems is to increase the number of covered lives. The mandatory enrollment of Medicaid beneficiaries into managed care products began in the system's service area, and its covered Medicaid lives increased rapidly from 10,000 to 40,000. Managed care enrollment in other products has also grown as the system has merged its IPA model and staff model HMOs. The strategy for growth is to retain multiple insurance options.

Market Influence in Mature Markets

In very competitive areas, the market continues to play a role in shaping system strategy and operations. For example, Friendly Hills HealthCare Network in LaHabra, Calif., has a national reputation as a well-run health care system. The California managed care market is certainly "mature." Since its inception, Friendly Hills has made a number of market-driven changes. For one, ownership and governance have shifted: Recently Friendly Hills' parent, Caremark, was acquired by MedPartners, Inc. The delivery system, too, has changed—enrollment in Friendly Hills increased from 100,000 to 400,000 covered lives in January 1996 when Caremark acquired 29 medical clinics previously owned by CIGNA (Friendly Hills 1996; Brown and Mayer 1997, 7–34).

CASE 6-5: BUILDING PRIMARY CARE CAPACITY

Integrated systems use both external standards and subjective judgment to determine the number and mix of providers. This example describes the approaches to primary care capacity taken by Lovelace Health Systems in New Mexico, Duke University Medical Center & Health System in North Carolina, and Partners HealthCare System in Massachusetts.

Lovelace Health Systems

Lovelace Health Systems is located in Albuquerque. The origins of Lovelace can be traced to the establishment of a group practice in the 1920s. In the 1970s, top leaders realized that excellence in specialty care would not guarantee referrals from primary care physicians who were unattached to the Lovelace Clinic. To develop its own primary care capability, Lovelace created a department of family practice. Initially, all family practice physicians were located in the central clinic in Albuquerque; later, some practitioners were moved 70 miles away to Santa Fe. Eventually, Lovelace set up departments of pediatrics and general internal medicine, and urgent care centers were integrated into the primary care programs (Ottensmeyer 1995).

Duke University Medical Center & Health System

Like Lovelace, Duke University Medical Center & Health System in Durham, N.C., realized that clinical excellence in tertiary and specialty care would not guarantee its future. Duke's early efforts to enhance primary care included acquisition of physicians in private practice, formal integration of family medicine physicians into the faculty practice plan, and administrative restructuring to give appropriate recognition to primary care.

Partners HealthCare System

Partners HealthCare System in Boston, the parent of Massachusetts General Hospital and Brigham and Women's Hospital, identified eastern Massachusetts as its target market. By the year 2000, the system expects to manage 1.5 to 2 million covered lives, of which 600,000 would be capitated. A related organization, Partners Community HealthCare, Inc. (PCHI) divided the geographic area into regional service organizations (RSOs). PCHI anticipated that 850 to 900 primary care physicians would be needed to meet enrollee needs across all RSOs (Montague 1995; Zane 1996).

CASE 6-6: COMBINING NOT-FOR-PROFIT AND FOR-PROFIT COMPONENTS

Some systems combine not-for-profit with for-profit entities. These hybrid organizations "offer the strength, speed, and capital of proprietaries, along with the strong values, stability, and community orientation of the mission-driven organization" (Flower 1996). Two examples are Tulane University Medical Center in Louisiana, and Methodist Health Care System in Texas.

Tulane University Medical Center

At Tulane University Medical Center, Columbia/HCA paid $132 million for 80 percent of the ownership of the hospital and clinics in 1995. The hospital became for-profit, but the 300 physicians remained faculty employees of Tulane University, a not-for-profit institution. Although contractual agreements between Columbia/ HCA and Tulane allowed a syndication that would have offered physicians investment opportunities, in 1997, Tulane University rejected such a plan for fear of jeopardizing its tax-exempt status (Japsen 1997).

Methodist Health Care System

Methodist Health Care System in San Antonio was created by the collaboration of Southwest Texas Methodist Hospital and smaller Columbia/HCA hospitals. The system is run by top leaders of Methodist Hospital, and there are Methodist chaplains. Also, system goals reflect Methodist Hospital ideals. Methodist Hospital has the ability to extricate itself from the arrangement under certain conditions, sell out at the acquisition price for several years, and deny the use of the Methodist name. The advantages to Methodist are the ability to retire debt and to apply a portion of the proceeds to the not-for-profit foundation for community uses.

CASE 6-7: COMBINATION VERSUS SEPARATION OF HEALTH CARE DELIVERY AND FINANCING

No rules of thumb indicate whether health care delivery and financing should be combined in integrated systems. Much depends on the characteristics of specific markets and organizations. Indecision, however, is not advisable. The following examples describe the approaches of different systems.

Fallon Healthcare System

For many years, the Fallon Healthcare System (described in case 6-1) thrived, grew in enrollment, provided high-quality care, and achieved its financial goals. By 1996, however, the competitive marketplace in New England had changed. The health plan component of the Fallon system no longer had the lowest premium. It was competing with large regional plans, many of which had been able to reduce their premiums. Internally, Fallon's ownership of its own health plan was perceived as a mixed blessing. In some respects, developing relationships with other plans was becoming more difficult because Fallon had already integrated both the delivery and financing of care (Podbielski 1996).

Mercy Health System

Mercy Health System, a vertically integrated rural health care system with 28 locations in southern Wisconsin and northern Illinois, has taken a different perspective. That system has its own insurance product, MercyCare Health Plans, and believes strongly that the symbiosis of delivery system and health plan will enable it to control its own destiny (Bea 1995).

Henry Ford Health System

Some integrated health care systems fall somewhere between the extremes; they neither seek out nor avoid the combination of delivery and financing. These systems generally are provider dominated and capable of juggling special insurance relationships through multiple contracts with other plans. Henry Ford Health System in Detroit, for example, owns the Health Alliance Plan, which accounts for a large share of the total number of the system's patients and gross revenue. System relationships with health plans other than its own are important, however, and Henry Ford has contracts with many other managed care plans and insurers.

Duke University Medical Center & Health System

Duke University Medical Center & Health System has taken a similar approach. Duke's relationship with NYLCare (formerly New York Life/Sanus) is special. The insurer and Duke undertook a joint venture in a new plan for university employees and in a commercial plan that is offered statewide. The partnership has enabled DUMC to rapidly learn how to manage patients in a capitated environment, and has also enabled NYLCare to incorporate outcomes of its experience with Duke into its health plans in other locations. Yet Duke maintains contractual relationships with many other health plans and employers (see chapter 7).

Graduate Health System and Advocate Health Care

Two systems that once linked delivery and financing but have divested themselves of their health plans are the Graduate Health System (GHS) in Philadelphia (now part of Allegheny Health, Education, and Research Foundation), and Advocate Health Care in Park Ridge, Ill. Hospital-based GHS had owned the Greater Atlantic Health System HMO, the third largest health plan in Philadelphia. In late 1995, it sold the plan and its other for-profit subsidiaries to reduce the hospitals' debt burden and increase the number of covered lives (Cramer and Kmetz 1995). Advocate Health Care's decision to sell its insurance subsidiary, Health Direct, was based on its desire to concentrate on the challenges of strengthening its delivery system (Votz and Cochrane 1996).

CASE 6-8: COMPETING SYSTEMS THAT COLLABORATE TO IMPROVE COMMUNITY HEALTH

Although integrated health care systems can use community health and advocacy as a competitive advantage, in some places competing systems collaborate for the good of the community at large (Zablocki 1996).

In South Bend, Ind., the Council of Clinics was formed by competitors Memorial Hospital and Health System, Ancilla Health Care, St. Joseph Medical Center, and Indiana Health Centers.

In Austin, Tex., the Health Partnership 2000 (HP2000) includes two major health systems, Seton Healthcare Network and Columbia/St. David's Health Care System, as well as the Austin/Travis County Health and Human Services Department, the HIV Planning Council, the Minority Health Network, and the Travis County Medical Society.

In Portland, Ore., the Oregon Health Systems in Collaboration is formally incorporated as a 501c(3) not-for-profit organization. Systems that collaborate are Kaiser Permanente's Northwest Division, Legacy Health System, Providence Health System in Oregon, Blue Cross/Blue Shield of Oregon, the Oregon Health Division, the Multnomah County Health Department, and the Oregon Health Sciences University.

CASE 6-9: PHILOSOPHICAL COMMITMENT TO INTEGRATED HEALTH CARE

Different organizations that come together to create an integrated health care system bring individual philosophies that are reflected in mission and goals, governance and structure, leadership and decision making, communications, and organizational culture. As a system they must build on what they have and create a new system culture.

Henry Ford Health System in Detroit has evolved from a hospital to a vertically integrated health system. By 1997, the system included owned as well as joint venture hospitals; more than 1,000 physicians organized into a multispecialty group practice and another 1,800 affiliated private-practice physicians; the full continuum of care, including ambulatory care clinics, long-term care, and home care, a mixed model health plan, and health and lifestyle services (Angell 1997).

Over the years, Henry Ford has identified and dealt with a number of problems related to forming a system. These include but are not limited to governance and management, physician mix, physician role in management, and improvement in clinical integration. For example, the corporate structure replaced 22 separate corporations that had functioned separately and competed for attention and resources. A streamlined management structure replaced nine layers. Prior to the creation of a medical group for employed physicians, physicians preferred working in small groups to working with a large organization. Before the implementation of specific programs to foster clinical integration, specialists and primary care physicians had not worked well together (Nighswander 1994).

An ongoing challenge has been the integration of clinical care across the entire system. The system has developed a major performance measure initiative, the Consortium Research on Indicators of System Performance. System researchers work continuously to develop appropriate and comprehensive measures for vertically integrated health systems that will provide a picture of "system performance" and enable Henry Ford to monitor its progress on an ongoing basis.

CASE 6-10: CHANGING CULTURE

Many of the country's most thoughtful systems executives believe that attention to change in the system's culture predicts success or failure. Managing culture change involves discussions of vision, values, and new behaviors; and rewards must be consistent with all of these. According to experienced systems leaders, changing culture takes from 3 to 10 years. The experiences of Henry Ford Health System in Michigan and Fairview Hospital and Healthcare Services in Minnesota provide two examples of managing change.

Henry Ford Health System

Henry Ford Health System in Detroit is used as an example throughout this book because of its many accomplishments over the years. Philosophical commitment to integration, physician leadership, and attention to quality are only three of those successes. Perhaps less well known is the work it has done on its values and attitudes—its culture.

At the point in its history when it had assembled the elements of a regional network, trustees and senior leaders at Henry Ford decided that the network's transformation to a system depended on its ability to create a single system culture to replace those of the previously separate organizations. The task was not easy (Wittrup, Sahney, and Warden 1994).

Although the separate components had legally come together, each organization and the departments within it remained financially responsible for their own bottom line. With respect to direct employer contracting, payers were interested in such relationships, but the system was ill equipped to respond.

To address the culture issue, Henry Ford adopted TQM, enhanced communication, and involved physicians in systemwide integration. As a philosophy of management, TQM had the potential to provide people throughout the system with a common language and way to approach their daily work. Therefore a systemwide TQM program (not a pilot) was implemented. With respect to communication, new strategies included creation of a chairman's council, a governance department that provided staff support to all boards, a system nominating committee, CEO Briefing (a newsletter), a three-year rolling planning process, senior organizational teams, an annual board retreat, and monthly meetings. Finally, physicians were well integrated into many operational and governance functions.

Despite all these efforts, in the minds of its own leaders, Henry Ford believes its attempts to change its culture must continue to develop so the culture permeates all layers of the organization.

Fairview Hospital and Healthcare Services

Although Fairview Hospital and Healthcare Services in Minneapolis has made many market-driven changes to remain competitive (case 6-12), it has also made a system commitment to defining and reinforcing its core values. In the words of the president and CEO, "it is important not to throw the baby out with the bath water" (Norling and Pashley 1995).

The process of identifying core values, making recommendations, and implementing them has extended over several years. It began with the appointment of a 20-member employee task force representing the various Fairview organizations. Representatives included middle managers, supervisors, team leaders, and front-line employees. The group identified core values, sought feedback and confirmation from peers, and revised and refined its initial list. Top leadership requested a stronger emphasis on Lutheran heritage. Additional suggestions were provided by 11 focus groups representing individuals associated with but not employed by Fairview. The list of core values was also tested with patients. The four core values selected were compassion, dignity, integrity, and service.

Following the identification of those values, the task force specified behaviors that would or would not support each value (Kennedy 1996). For example, behaviors that would support compassion included intuitive sensitivity to others' needs and attentive listening to patients and coworkers without providing advice. Again, the task force tested its work, this time with two patient focus groups.

Prior to making recommendations, the task force identified factors that might facilitate or restrain the implementation of a program to reinforce core values. Positive factors included individuals' dedication, and their desire to do a good job and contribute to the organization; management commitment to CQI and desire to minimize conflict; physician and board support and overall organizational commitment to CQI. Restraining forces included individual apathy and lack of commitment; skepticism about the long-term implementation of the program and long-term management commitment; confusion and fear; turf issues; deficiencies in skills needed to make the program work; cumbersome decision-making characterized by decentralization; and strong emphasis on bottom-line financial performance that could potentially deter emphasis on values.

The task force made 12 recommendations and suggested both a structural and synergistic approach. The structural aspect involved design of work groups that would directly tackle recommendations. The synergistic approach encouraged the merging and reshaping of implementation activities into new initiatives. Strengthening plans grouped various activities into four groups: communication, modeling behavior, education and training, and revising systems.

Fairview learned several important lessons during the implementation process (Norling and Pashley 1995). First, the organization did not move as a single entity; different parts learned at different speeds. Second, interest in the emphasis on core values came in waves that ebbed and flowed. Different interest levels did not mean loss of interest; rather, they reflected attention to day-to-day priorities. One effective way to maintain interest over time was to identify a single individual as a resource to be contacted with questions. Third, many managers were initially skeptical.

Future challenges relating to emphasis on core values include impact of core values on collaboration with other organizations, on relationships with affiliated physicians who are not owned by the system, and, potentially, on clinical care.

CASE 6-11: CLEAR PURPOSE AND VISION

Clarity of purpose and vision is imperative for integrated health care systems regardless of size and location of the system. Baylor Health Care System in Texas and Copley Health System in Vermont are examples of systems with such vision.

Baylor Health Care System

In the early 1990s, the Dallas/Fort Worth area lacked the market forces that often inspire radical change in health care financing and delivery. Although system leaders at Baylor Health Care System felt no urgent pressure, they looked elsewhere in the country and decided that a fully integrated system was the best long-term strategy for Baylor University Medical Center and the community medical centers. However, many barriers to creating such a system included pride in past success and aversion to change, traditional hospital focus, local governance, and lack of consensus on core values (Shortell and others 1996).

A thoughtful planning process focusing on Baylor as an integrated system began in 1994. The System Integration Action Team was created to look at the system as a whole. Headed by the senior executive vice president and chief operating officer, the group of 28 employees and physicians met for more than a year. It focused on seven core processes: managing patient illness across the continuum; wellness; coordination of member education and access to care; development, updating, and communicating system strategies; capturing market; assessing and managing risk; and management of resources that would support core processes. The target date for achieving integration objectives that grew out of this planning process was January 1, 1997 (Allison 1997).

Copley Health System

Copley Health System in Morrisville, Vt., is an integrated delivery system that provides care for 26,000 people in 16 rural Vermont towns located in the northwestern part of the state. Unlike other systems that emphasize structure rather than purpose, Copley has concentrated on its goals from the beginning. Its small size (54 beds) and nonurban location have not been deterrents. The mission statement adopted in 1991 emphasizes wellness and prevention, improvement of health status, provision of the highest quality of care to the sick and injured, and provision of care regardless of ability to pay. An important aspect of that mission is to act as a community resource (Roberts 1996).

Formal and informal structural arrangements support the system's strategic intent. The parent company, Copley Health System, was formed in 1985. Since that time, there has been a clear intent to keep people out of the hospital by developing diverse activities. Primary care is provided by physicians and midlevel practitioners. Copley Hospital provides primary and some secondary inpatient acute care (for example, CT scan, intensive care, and emergency care).

Copley alone can neither provide the full continuum of care to the population that it serves nor accept financial risk through capitation. Therefore, it has partnered with a tertiary facility, Fletcher Allen Health Care, and developed strong working relationships with components of care that it does not provide, such as long-term and home care.

CASE 6-12: STRONG PHYSICIAN LEADERSHIP

Physician integration and strong leadership involves at least five components: emphasis on management of care by primary care physicians and other providers; physician representation in governance and administration; physician involvement in operations, particularly care management across the continuum; physician acceptance of financial risk and alignment of physician and system financial incentives; and education and training for physicians that focuses on management of care; cost and quality; and leadership skills. This case describes Henry Ford Health System in Michigan, Fairview Hospital and Healthcare Services in Minnesota, Friendly Hills HealthCare Network in California, and North Shore Health System in Massachusetts.

Henry Ford Health System

Henry Ford Health System in Detroit has existed since Henry Ford Hospital was founded in 1915—long enough to provide important insights into the evolutionary way in which a system that was once hospital-dominated has addressed physician leadership.

The system has both salaried and affiliated physician providers. The Henry Ford Medical Group physicians are salaried with performance bonuses; the community physicians affiliated with the system are compensated according to a variety of reimbursement methods.

Throughout its growth, the physician component of the system has experienced and addressed several major problems. Salaried physicians were accustomed to functioning in small specialty-specific groups. At the outset, they had difficulty relating to a larger organization. To address this problem, employed physicians were organized into a single medical group where physician leadership was an important component.

Henry Ford has experienced an imbalance in the ratio of primary care and specialty physicians. Even when system growth became aggressive, the ratio of primary care to specialty physicians was below the stated goal of 50:50 (Schultz 1995). To correct the ratio and make the delivery system more responsive to managed care needs, Henry Ford developed two physician recruitment strategies. Its long-term strategy was collaboration with Case Western Reserve University School of Medicine in Cleveland to develop a generalist track in training and residency programs. Its short-term approach was to recruit primary care physicians already in practice by offering a variety of affiliation options, including but not limited to contracting to provide specific services to HMO patients, employment by a Henry Ford hospital, and salaried membership in the Henry Ford multispecialty group practice.

Correcting the ratio of primary care to specialist physicians was only part of the primary care problem. Adding primary care capacity to the system would have positive results only if clinical and administrative staff understood how to relate to primary care physicians. To deal with this issue and others, Henry Ford developed the Managed Care College "to educate staff on the intricacies of managed care" (Managed care education 1996). The program had the following three strategies:

- Emphasis on the process, not the structure of managing care
- Concentration on identification of the population's most common medical needs
- Determination of the most efficient and medically prudent ways to meet patient needs

The Managed Care College has expanded to educate the entire Henry Ford Health System.

Fairview Hospital and Healthcare Services

In the early 1990s, the organization that is now Fairview Hospital and Healthcare Services in Minneapolis–St. Paul faced external pressures in both private and public sectors. Physicians met the challenge, and with strong leadership, have made an important difference.

In the private sector, a purchasing coalition, now comprising 23 employers including the state of Minnesota and representing 115,000 covered lives, selected a limited number of systems from which it would purchase care. The Fairview physicians were not selected in the competitive bidding process. Among their shortcomings were a loose structure, inadequate quality improvement planning and implementation, and inadequate integration among physicians and between physicians and hospital (Burmaster 1995 and 1997).

Faced with the loss of a significant amount of business, the Fairview physicians reorganized themselves into the Fairview Physician Associates (FPA), a network of independent and employed physicians that would function and contract as a multispecialty group and as a care system, assuming responsibility for improvement of the health status of the people it served. By 1997, FPA included 550 independent and 150 employed physicians; 300 of that number were primary care practitioners. The governing board included four primary care and two specialist physicians, eight representatives of the community, the FPA president, the Fairview Hospital CEO, and a representative of the clinic administrator. FPA and Fairview Hospital have developed a partnership relationship that has enabled them to respond to the needs of both employers and health plans (Burmaster 1997).

Friendly Hills HealthCare Network

The Friendly Hills HealthCare Network in LaHabra, Calif., was formed in 1968, when Friendly Hills began as a family practice–based group practice. Both structure and ownership have changed, and Friendly Hills is now an equity model integrated delivery system owned by MedPartners, Inc. That company bought Caremark, previously the parent of Friendly Hills. The following description of physician involvement predates the new arrangement.

Physician leadership at Friendly Hills has been strong since the outset. The president/CEO is a physician, and the senior vice president of medical affairs reported directly to him. The organization chart shown in figure 6-4 illustrates the division of responsibilities. Three line medical directors managed care across all regions and were responsible for CIGNA family practice, pediatrics, and obstetrics/ gynecology; Friendly Hills Medical Group (FHMG); and CIGNA medical subspecialties. Three staff medical directors were responsible for quality management, medical education and consulting, and utilization management. Both primary and subspecialty care were managed across regions to promote efficient scheduling and coverage. Department chairs made recommendations to the medical directors but did not make final decisions.

Although it has prided itself on strong medical management, as it grew and changed, Friendly Hills encountered difficult challenges (Brown and Mayer 1997, 7–34). For example, in January 1996, Caremark/Friendly Hills purchased 29 practices previously owned by CIGNA. Overnight, enrollment quadrupled from 100,000 to 400,000, and physicians from group and staff model backgrounds had the opportunity to work together in a new organization.

Culturally, there was a significant difference between the physicians who had been practicing in the FHMG and the physicians who had worked in the staff model CIGNA practices. FHMG owned itself. Physicians were accustomed to self-governance and decision making by peers. In contrast, physicians in the CIGNA practices

FIGURE 6-4.   Friendly Hills HealthCare Network—Medical Management

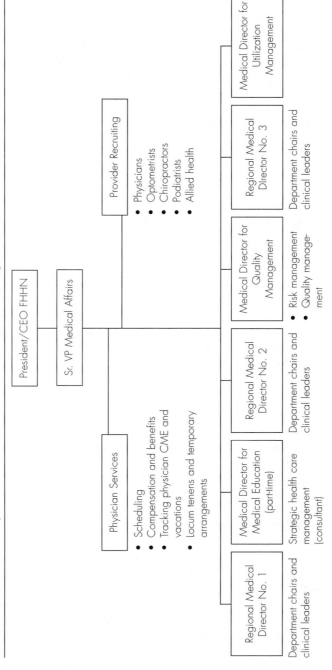

Source: Mayer, T. 1997. Interview by author. Friendly Hills HealthCare Foundation, Whittier, Calif., 25 April.

were accustomed to decision making by the insurer, their employer and owner.

To integrate the FHMG and CIGNA physicians into a cohesive single unit, the senior vice president of medical affairs followed a number of carefully phased steps (Mayer 1997). First, medical leadership was shared. Three of the six medical directors were selected from the CIGNA practices, and the other three came from FHMG. For CIGNA physicians to become part of the new professional corporation, they had to agree to a financial arrangement that guaranteed only 80 percent of their salary. The remaining 20 percent was based on performance criteria such as productivity and resource management.

Another step was the selection of department chairs by the medical directors. Each department chair designated a clinical leader responsible for care in each of four regions. Department chairs were responsible for standardizing work ethic and compensation. Chairs made recommendations to medical directors, and the latter made decisions. Chairs supervised the nomination and election of three CIGNA physicians to the board of the new medical group.

Representatives of each department nominated by department chairs sat on the compensation committee. Working with the senior vice president of medical affairs and three medical directors, this new committee determined year-end bonuses for the group and designed performance criteria for the next year. Throughout the process, communication was frequent and open.

North Shore Health System

The North Shore Health System in Salem, Mass., is an integrated health care organization that is also part of the Partners HealthCare System. Traditionally, physicians practicing in Salem and surrounding communities were not particularly well organized. Participation in governance and medical management was limited to token representation on the hospital board, medical staff activities, and health plan–specific medical management.

The formation of North Shore and its formal linkage to Partners Community HealthCare, Inc. (PCHI) has been heavily influenced by physician leadership (Fallon 1996). Physicians are involved in governance, medical management, and strategic planning. North Shore has a physician president. The 16-person board includes eight physicians, of whom five specialize in primary care. With respect to medical management, North Shore has received delegated review authority from several risk plans. The approach to modifying physician behavior is positive, not punitive. Twenty-five physicians participate in medical management, thus encouraging involvement beyond a handful of committed few. On-site physicians handle referral management, and claims denial is minimal. When problems in the management of care surface, they are addressed in educational sessions. In fact, financial incentives encourage physician participation in education. NSHS supports its medical management with both homegrown practice guidelines and externally developed protocols modified for local use.

North Shore physicians also play an important role in guiding and governing Partners Community HealthCare, Inc., the larger system of which it is part. In fact, many of North Shore's accomplishments are models for physicians in other communities. North Shore and others vigorously supported the significant involvement of community physicians, many of whom specialize in primary care, in the governance structure and committees of PCHI. As a result, the PCHI network has won acceptance outside the academic medical center community and has become attractive to payers.

CASE 6-13: ALIGNMENT OF FINANCIAL INCENTIVES AND REWARDS FOR SYSTEM PERFORMANCE

All integrated health care systems must align financial incentives and rewards to recognize system performance. If financial arrangements are inconsistent with system long-term goals or if there are mixed financial incentives within a given system, progress and success are obstructed. Three important concepts are willingness to accept financial risk for the cost and utilization of care, consistency of financial incentives, and financial rewards for system performance. The system described in this case is Samaritan Health System in Phoenix.

At Samaritan Health System, compensation recognizes and rewards system behavior. The human resources development has gone several steps further, making sure that employee evaluations, training, development, hiring, orientation, and communication are consistent with system cohesion and customer service (Moore 1996).

Phoenix is a competitive managed care market. More than 70 percent of the population is covered by managed care. Samaritan Health System has 30 percent of that 70 percent, so the stakes are high indeed.

The components of Samaritan Health System include Good Samaritan Regional Medical Center (642-bed tertiary facility), Maryvale Samaritan Medical Center (256 beds), Thunderbird Samaritan Medical Center (235 beds), Desert Samaritan Medical Center (414 beds), two outlying hospitals, six primary care facilities, five behavioral health centers, two skilled nursing facilities, and a 350,000 member HMO. The system is also involved in a full-asset merger with HealthPartners of Southern Arizona in Tucson; that new entity is expected to be called Integra Health System.

As the Samaritan Health System has grown, employee compensation has been one of the issues upon which senior management has concentrated. The system's vice president for human resources and a team of 18 people from throughout the system took on the challenge of "system infrastructure." Their goal was to develop a compensation system that rewarded results and did not flow from controlled resources.

As the team began its work on compensation, it discovered that pay was not the only issue; performance was also important. Did employees take initiative and were they rewarded for doing so? Did people go out of their way to respond to patient concerns? How did employees relate to their colleagues? Did people work on behalf of the system or just their own department or institution?

The work of the team became more complicated. If behaviors that emphasized system goals and patients were desirable, how would Samaritan teach its employees what it wanted them to do? Education and training as well as compensation needed revision.

The performance appraisal portion of the Samaritan plan ties compensation to performance. Employees are rated as developing, competent, or masters level. Jobs are broken down into functional competencies (technical skills needed to perform jobs) and core competencies (behavioral portion of performance management). One of the most important questions asked in the core competency portion of the appraisal is, "In his/her daily actions, does the employee contribute to the success of Samaritan Health System?"

CASE 6-14: FOCUS ON HEALTHY COMMUNITIES

Integrated health care systems must pay attention to the community as a major customer. There is a potential symbiosis between integrated health care and healthy communities that some but not all systems recognize.

Even those systems that accept their responsibility to the community define the word differently. Community may mean individual enrollees of a system, the community at large (including but not limited to system enrollees), and those two groups as well as people who cannot afford to pay for health insurance.

This case describes the approach to community health taken by three systems: Group Health Cooperative in Washington; Laurel Health System in Pennsylvania; and Appalachian Regional Healthcare in Kentucky, Virginia, and West Virginia.

Group Health Cooperative

Group Health Cooperative (GHC) in Seattle is one of the country's oldest HMOs and the sixth largest not-for-profit plan in the country (Southwick 1996). It is a staff model plan with 550,000 members. The delivery system includes 30 primary care medical centers, two hospitals, six specialty centers, one skilled nursing facility, and a home care facility. GHC has contractual relationships with 48 hospitals. One thousand physicians are affiliated exclusively with the plan, and another 2,500 have contractual relationships. Recent initiatives include a joint venture with Virginia Mason Medical Center and a "merger-like partnership" with Kaiser Permanente's Northwest Division.

GHC broadly defines the community for which it is responsible. With its history of consumerism, the plan is committed to community service and social responsibility. It collaborates with other providers and seeks ways to enhance existing efforts in order to understand and meet the needs of underserved populations at risk. Employees, staff, and consumer members are encouraged to participate in volunteer activities.

Within the "community" of its own enrollees, GHC has initiated a number of programs targeted at particular disease categories. Proactive care for diabetics is one of its priorities. GHC first identified 12,000 of its enrollees as diabetics who had two of the following three characteristics: elevated blood sugar, use of a hypoglycemic agent such as insulin, or actual diagnosis of diabetes through a hospital or clinic visit. A multidisciplinary team then identified desirable outcomes such as improvement in function and vision, decreased complications, improved control of blood pressure and blood sugar, and decreased amputation and ulceration.

Because so many diabetics see primary care providers, these physicians received both a "road map" to guide the provision of care and a team to support them. Team members included a certified diabetes educator, a nutritionist with expertise in diabetic issues, and others. Physicians and other team members could check each diabetic patient's progress by an on-line system.

Laurel Health System

System efforts to improve community health are not limited to large entities with many years of experience. In fact, smaller systems and rural systems with more circumscribed service areas often have a distinct advantage. Many of these systems have long histories of close collaboration with other health care and non-health-care organizations in an effort to respond to community needs.

An example is the Laurel Health System in Wellsboro, Penn. The focus for its assessment of community needs was Tioga County, which had 14,000 households. Partnerships between the health system, educational institutions, churches, insurers, lending institutions, the chamber of commerce, the American Association of Retired Persons, and county government enabled the group to understand and deal collectively with the problems it identified. Many of the participating partners contributed financial support; others provided labor and other resources (Sandrick 1995).

Appalachian Regional Healthcare

Appalachian Regional Healthcare (ARH) is an example of a rural integrated system with commitment to the community as customer. The not-for-profit system serves central Appalachian communities in Kentucky, Virginia, and West Virginia. The delivery system includes 11 hospitals ranging in size from 30 to more than 300 beds, primary care clinics, special programs (such as maternal and child health and mental health), and home care agencies/stores.

The mission of ARH reflects its community focus. The mission is "to provide high-quality health care and to conduct educational activities to promote the general health of the region [it serves] without regard to race, creed, religion, color, age, sex, national origin, or economic status." Communities offer an "opportunity to serve" (Appalachian Regional Healthcare 1995).

With the assistance of the Center for Rural Health at the University of Kentucky in Hazard, ARH has piloted a community decision-making (CDM) program designed to involve local communities in health care planning (Williams 1996). A "community encourager" was hired to assume the role of liaison between community and providers. After the encourager met with community representatives, representatives of different groups were selected to serve on a community health council. The encourager and the community health council held focus group meetings to assess needs; the meetings were followed up with direct mail. In a town meeting format, needs were posted, discussed, and prioritized. The health care system and other agencies then used hard data to determine the feasibility of suggested options. In Harlan County, Ky., work done by the CDM program resulted in a new emergency medical service within a relatively short time frame.

CASE 6-15: INFORMATION SYSTEMS AND INFORMATION TECHNOLOGY

Information systems and information technology (IS/IT) is essential to systems integration. When information systems and technology support an integrated system, clinicians, enrollees, and external purchasers all benefit. Nonetheless, there is an important caveat regarding IS/IT: It is a support function, not a solution.

This case describes the approaches to IS/IT taken by Advocate Health Care in Illinois, Allina Health System in Minnesota, and Graduate Health System in Pennsylvania.

Advocate Health Care

Advocate Health Care in Park Ridge, Ill., is the result of the 1995 merger of two hospital-based systems, Lutheran General Health System (LGHS) and Evangelical Health System (EHS). By early

1996, Advocate had 80 facilities/centers in the Chicago metropolitan area, and the geographic expansion created a difficult challenge for the building of systems infrastructure.

An important aspect of Advocate's IS/IT strategy for the combined organization was making sure that information available to administrators and clinicians provided "knowledge value" (Reep 1995). The two systems entered into the merger with different IS/IT capabilities. Faced with a choice of starting from zero or preserving some of its existing legacy computer applications, Advocate decided to build on what already existed. Plans for the Advocate IS system included uniform information distribution throughout the organization. There would be some open architecture systems (for example, Unix, Windows®, and Windows® 95) that allowed integration of various types of components.

Advocate's IS/IT planning effort was consistent with the system planning effort. Group-based IS/IT planning and vendor selection went well, and there was a balance between centralization and decentralization of IS/IT. Nonetheless, two of the difficult challenges that Advocate faced were integrating the cultures of different organizations and reinforcing a systemwide appreciation for information technology.

Allina Health System

The 1994 merger that created Allina Health System in Minneapolis brought together a health plan (Medica) and an integrated health services organization (HealthSpan). Allina's development of a systemwide IS/IT system was therefore tailored to an enterprise that combined health care delivery and financing.

Allina's IS/IT goals had a clinical focus: to provide connections across organizations, outstanding support to providers, and support/facilitation for clinical policy initiatives (Reep 1995). Both the health services system and the health plan had existing IS systems, including mainframe and minidistributed computing, multiple care applications at different hospitals, and multiple niche systems that had been developed in-house and outsourced.

Plans called for common applications for all hospitals, an Allina wide-area network), a systemwide data repository, access by multiple system customers, and systemwide scheduling. The use of telemedicine to link 22 remote sites in Minnesota and Wisconsin already connected rural and urban system components (Telemedicine 1996).

Allina developed rolling one-year IS/IT planning cycles. Thus IS/IT planning has time-specific targets but also evolves as the organization grows. The IS/IT vision is clear; strategy and tactics are expected to develop over time.

Graduate Health System

Graduate Health System (GHS), now part of Allegheny Health, Education, and Research Foundation, had headquarters in Philadelphia. The geographic area served by the system extended into suburban communities in Pennsylvania and New Jersey. The evolution of GHS began in the late 1980s. Graduate Hospital, a tertiary care hospital with research and teaching affiliations with the University of Pennsylvania Schools of Medicine and Dentistry, embarked on a strategy of building relationships with other hospitals and developing system infrastructure (Cramer and Kmetz 1995).

By 1995, GHS included hospitals, physicians, Founder's Healthcare, Inc. (which owned and operated physician practices), GHS Home Medical Services, Concorde Clinical Research, and more than a dozen for-profit subsidiaries that provided medical support activities, medical imaging, and other services. In addition, GHS operated the Greater Atlantic Health System HMO, the third largest plan in Philadelphia. The system also had been aggressive in Medicare and Medicaid risk contracting. (In 1995, GHS sold its HMO and other for-profit subsidiaries to Health Systems International [HSI] of California. A year later, it announced its intention to enter into negotiations with Allegheny.)

Like other urban markets, Greater Philadelphia was very competitive. The city was home to multiple academic medical centers that had developed linkages with one another and with community providers (Iglehart 1995). When GHS eventually linked with one of those major systems, it brought with it an unusual understanding of the importance of information systems and valuable experience.

GHS's long-term plans to leverage information technologies for competitive advantage had multiple components. In 1990 the system created a new position, corporate vice president for planning and technology. This system executive had broad responsibility for strategic planning, program development, and information technology, the goal of which was to guide all three on parallel tracks. Decision making for IS/IT was carefully thought out and involved both centralized IS staff and end-users.

GHS's early commitment to technological excellence resulted in a number of achievements (Cramer and Kmetz 1995). Using both fiberoptic and T1 lines and supports, the Ethernet wide area network supported many applications: computerized patient records (CPR), interactive video technology that extended the reach of teaching activities, systemwide materials management, financial and accounting systems, systemwide physician credentialing, human resources, E-mail, systemwide scheduling, and quality outcomes systems. Local area networks allowed the development of user-specific applications.

One of GHS's first applications, the CPR permitted the system to achieve numerous cost savings and clinical improvements. For example, the CPR permitted downsizing of several laboratories and increased use of the central laboratory at Graduate Hospital. Although the processing was done centrally, test results were available on line at the different user sites. The CPR also allowed cost savings in medical and surgical supplies. Clinical improvements resulting from the CPR impacted the pharmacy area and the analysis of practice patterns and outcomes. Graduate expected the CPR to facilitate managing care across the continuum.

Although GHS ownership changed in 1996, its IS/IT capability has remained strong. HSI, the California company that purchased GHS's HMO and other for-profit subsidiaries in 1995, is committed to IS excellence. That company is pilot-testing fourth-generation medical management that makes extensive clinical data available to providers, and the GHS hospitals and physicians are part of this test (HSI pioneers 1996).

CASE 6-16: COMMITMENT TO QUALITY

Attention to quality is an imperative for integrated health care systems. The challenge of quality in a systems context involves conceptualization, technical competence, and the ability to apply the results of quality assessment to ongoing quality improvement. This case describes the approaches to quality of two integrated systems in New Mexico: Lovelace Health Systems and Presbyterian Healthcare Services. Although both systems compete in the same market, they are structured differently. Consequently, each has developed a unique approach to quality.

Lovelace Health Systems

Lovelace Health Systems in Albuquerque is an integrated system that has evolved significantly over the past 20 years. It now combines both health care delivery and financing (Ottensmeyer 1995). Under the leadership of a strong physician group, Lovelace currently provides care for 200,000 people, of whom 70 percent (140,000) are enrolled in the Lovelace Health Plan. Since 1989, Lovelace has been strongly committed to total quality management.

The Lovelace organization comprises Lovelace Health Systems, the Lovelace Clinic Foundation, and the Lovelace Institutes. The delivery system includes a 200-physician group practice, a 325-bed hospital (Lovelace Medical Center Hospital), 15 primary care centers, and an affiliated network of 900 physicians and 12 hospitals (Friedman 1996; Cochrane 1996). In 1985, Lovelace was sold to a joint venture partnership including HCA and Equicorp. Since CIGNA's purchase of Equicorp in 1990, that insurer has owned Lovelace.

Because the Lovelace Clinic has played such an important role in the system's development, physicians have always been influential in governance and management. At the governance level, 50 percent of the parent organization's members are physicians: the system CEO, three clinic physicians, and the system chief medical officer. At the management level, four of seven senior managers are physicians. Physicians are influential throughout the system. In addition to those already mentioned, department chairs, section chiefs, the HMO medical director, and the directors of utilization review, TQM, and research play important roles.

Although Lovelace is a strong player in the Albuquerque market, competition is intense. For Lovelace to achieve its long-term enrollment target, it must outperform its competitors and create value for purchasers and enrollees. With this goal in mind, in 1992 Lovelace developed a list of quality indicators that could describe the system. These included patient satisfaction, health plan disenrollment, and staff turnover. Clearly missing from the list were clinical indicators other than the traditional ones of mortality, postoperative infections, and rates of cesarean section. Quality improvement activities existed throughout the system, but they were fragmented and unrelated to the organization's strategic objectives.

To correct its problems, Lovelace revised its approach to quality and developed a coordinated approach that incorporated primary and specialty care in both inpatient and outpatient settings. An important catalyst was marketplace interest in cost reduction and evidence of quality.

For Lovelace, relatively few conditions accounted for a large proportion of costs. Specifically, 80 percent of the costs could be attributed to 30 health conditions. LHS used an "episode of care" (EOC) approach to address these problems. It defined EOC as "all the services provided to a patient with a particular medical problem, within a specified period of time, across the continuum of care." The episode includes all aspects of care—prevention, access, assessment, treatment, and aftercare/follow-up (Friedman 1996).

The initial EOC effort resulted in the creation of nine teams that addressed diabetes, pediatric asthma, coronary artery disease, pregnancy/birth, low back pain, breast cancer, stroke, depression, and knee care. The nine areas were selected based on four criteria: high risk to patients, high volume within the system, high variation in provider practice patterns, and high cost. To support the effort, Lovelace restructured its quality management department. Now called the department of clinical practice improvement and quality management, it supports the different EOC teams in their efforts. Early in 1996, Lovelace went one step further. Lovelace Healthcare Innovations, Inc. signed an agreement to develop and validate 30 disease management programs (now called platforms of care) for marketing by Greenstone Healthcare Solutions (Phillips 1996).

Each episode or platform of care program costs between $200,000 and $500,000. The return on investment is measured by looking at practice efficiencies and lower rates of disease complications. Quality of life and patient satisfaction are also measured. Physicians receive a report card for each EOC so that they can see patients' progress across an established outcome parameter.

Several tools have facilitated the development of the EOCs. Each development team includes not only physicians and other caregivers, but a new type of specialist called a clinical practice improvement coach. He or she performs many of the functions previously done separately, including quality assurance; risk, utilization, and case management; discharge planning; and education. Advances in information systems facilitate the EOC program, and providers have access to information that incorporates input from multiple databases.

Lovelace's disease management initiative is tremendously important to the system. To become a member of the Lovelace Physician Group, a physician must assume responsibility for clinical practice improvement as well as for patient care.

Presbyterian Healthcare Services

Although Lovelace Health Systems receives much publicity for attention to quality, the achievements of a competing system are also impressive. Presbyterian Healthcare Services (PHS) provides care to 225,000 people in Albuquerque and 15 rural communities. Tertiary referrals come from a larger service area.

Structurally, PHS includes three hospitals (of which one is a 550-bed tertiary care center), five family health centers, an HMO, and a medical staff of 650 that provides care in multiple facilities. PHS describes its medical staff as "fiercely independent, specialty oriented, internally competitive, and competing with three other local integrated systems" (Bader 1994). The PHS network is not a legal entity. Because a state tax law would require a medical foundation to pay a state tax of 5.75 percent gross receipts, the affiliation has remained loose.

Although PHS is structured very differently from Lovelace, it too is committed to quality. The creation of the network in 1990 involved formal recognition of the role that physicians would play and the importance of the quality imperative. Quality was built into PHS in five ways: physician involvement and empowerment, customer focus, credentialing, commitment to CQI, and recognition of the need for cultural transformation.

Physician Involvement and Empowerment   Physicians are formally involved in governance and management in multiple ways. The network board acts in an advisory capacity to the PHS system board. It includes 15 physicians, an administrator, the PHS president, and the PHS board chairman. The physician management committee is composed of an elected physician leader and lead physicians from each group practice and facility. It meets every two weeks to discuss policy issues that extend across practice sites. Three network sub-boards represent hospital-based, office-based, and specialty physicians. The network selection committee evaluates and recommends physicians for network participation based on preestablished criteria. The information systems steering committee also includes physicians and reports to the system board. This physician representation also includes three physician vice presidents and nine part-time physician program directors who manage service lines.

Customer Focus   An important component of PHS's quality efforts is its focus on customers, including both network physicians and patients. The system emphasizes "organized care" based on internally driven definitions of quality, rather than "managed care" that many physicians perceive as imposing standards from outside the system. Organized care means voluntarily coming together to manage the system and accept financial risk for a population over time.

Credentialing   Physicians who wish to join the PHS network are credentialed according to criteria set by the network selection committee. There is no membersip fee, but potential members must participate in an orientation. The application asks questions about quality improvement, patient satisfaction, compatibility with network practice, board certification, and continuing medical education. Potential members are also asked about participation in quality initiatives and cost reduction efforts. Physicians who join the network must participate in CQI activities.

Cultural Transformation   PHS's emphasis on quality is new to many of the physicians in the network. Therefore, leadership believes that a cultural transformation will be necessary to make the quality efforts effective.

CASE 6-17: FOCUS ON MARKET-DRIVEN VALUE

Organizations and individuals in integrated health care systems tend to focus on internal issues: structure, governance, financing, and management. They generally do not look outside the system at the market that will buy or reject what they have to offer.

Examples of systems that pay attention to market-driven customer value are Henry Ford Health System in Michigan, Dartmouth-Hitchcock Northern Region in New England, and Mercy Health Services in Michigan. Each of these systems has identified its own list of important customer-specific measures. Table 6-1 includes these measures to provide readers with suggested features to measure.

TABLE 6-1. Important Measures of Customer Value in Three
Integrated Health Care Systems

Henry Ford Health System	Dartmouth-Hitchcock Northern Region	Mercy Health Services
External customer satisfaction	Access	Clinical quality
Clinical process/ outcomes	Patient satisfaction	Service quality
Financial performance	Patient-specific functional health status	Organizational capability and adaptability of staff
Philanthropy	Community image as perceived by community residents	Cost reduction
Community divided	Employee satisfaction	Community health care
Growth (market)	Management process	At-risk population programs
Business strategic advantage	Referring physician satisfaction	
Innovation	Volume of services	
Internal customer satisfaction (employees)	Profitability	
Academic endeavors (research and education)	Research	
	Information systems (as rated by employees)	

References

Allison, J. 1997. Interview by author. Baylor Health Care System, Dallas, 26 March.

American Hospital Association. 1993. Case study: Rehobeth McKinley Christian Health Care Services. In *Working from within: Integrating rural health care*. Chicago: American Hospital Association.

Angell, D. 1997. Interview by author. Henry Ford Health System, Detroit, 27 March.

Appalachian Regional Healthcare. 1995. Public relations material.

Bader, B. S. 1994. Visionary systems design quality into their integrated care networks. Integrated system profile: Presbyterian Healthcare Services, Albuquerque, New Mexico. In *Successful Strategies for Building an Integrated Hospital/Physician Healthcare System*. Rockville, Md.: Bader & Associates.

Baker, W. L., and M. Dubree. 1996. Vanderbilt University and Clinic: Retooling medical care through collaborative organizational design. In *Redesigning healthcare delivery,* edited by P. Boland. Berkeley, Calif.: Boland Healthcare.

Bea, J. 1995. Mercy Health System. Presentation at Integrated Healthcare Symposium, Aspen, Colo., 25–26 September.

Brown, H. P., and T. Mayer. 1997. Moving from physician-hospital organizations to integrated delivery systems. In *Hospital strategies in managed care,* edited by J. Burns and M. Sipkoff. New York: Faulkner & Gray, Inc.

Burmaster, R. 1995. Fairview Physician Associates. Presentation at Integrated Healthcare Symposium, Aspen, Colo., 25–26 September.

———. 1997. Interview by author. Fairview Physician Associates, Minneapolis, 4 April.

Cochrane, J. 1996. Scenes from Aspen. Lovelace: A physician-driven integrated health care system. *Integrated Health Care Report* 6–7 (September).

Cramer, H., and J. Kmetz. 1995. Interview by author. Graduate Health System, Philadelphia, 18 September.

Fallon, J. A. 1996. Interview by author. North Shore Health System, Salem, Mass., 18 October.

Flower, J. 1996. Pride and prejudice. *Healthcare Forum Journal* 39: 26–34 (March/April).

Friedman, N. 1996. Diabetes and managed care: The Lovelace Health Systems' episode of care program. *Managed Care Quarterly* 4: 43–49 (winter).

Friendly Hills HealthCare Network. 1996. Duke University Medical Center site visit, 6 May.

Henry Ford Health System. 1995. *Business and Health* 13 (12): Special Section (December).

Hensley, S. 1997a. Exceeding expectations: Execs of 1-year-old Premier detail ambitious plans. *Modern Healthcare* 27 (6): 20–21 (10 February).

———. 1997b. Premier unit to test alliance's clout. *Modern Healthcare* 27 (18): 3, 16 (5 May).

HSI pioneers new data system. 1996. *Integrated Health Report* 11–12 (September).

Iglehart, J. K. 1995. Academic medical centers enter the market: The case of Philadelphia. *New England Journal of Medicine* 333 (15): 1019–1023 (12 October).

Japsen, B. 1997. Columbia rejected in La. *Modern Healthcare* 27 (17): 6 (28 April).

Kanter, R. M., and B. A. Stein. 1993. *Strategic alliances: Some lessons from experience.* Cambridge, Mass.: Goodmeasure, Inc.

Keener, S. R., J. W. Baker, and G. P. Mays. 1997. Providing public health services through an integrated delivery system. *Quality Management in Health Care* 5: 27–34.

Kennedy, M. 1996. Creating a new postmerger culture. *Health System Leader* 3 (5): 4–11 (June).

Managed care education can be internal process. 1996. *Hospital Managed Care Strategies* 4: 10–11 (January).

Mayer, T. 1997. Interview by author. Friendly Hills HealthCare Foundation, Whittier, Calif., 5 May.

Montague, J. 1995. When the smoke clears. *Hospitals and Health Networks* 69: 65–68 (5 February).

Moore, J. D. 1996. Samaritan's revolution: New pay model aims to overhaul how workers think. *Modern Healthcare* 26 (31): 27–30 (29 July).

Nighswander, A. 1994. *Integrated health care delivery: A blueprint for action*. St. Paul, Minn.: InterStudy Publications.

Norling, R. A., and S. Pashley. 1995. Identifying and strengthening core values. *Managed Care Quarterly* 3: 11–28.

Nurkin, H. A. 1995. The creation of a multiorganizational health care alliance: The Charlotte-Mecklenburg Hospital Authority. In *Partners for the dance: Forming strategic alliances in health care*, by A. D. Kaluzny, H. S. Zuckerman, and T. C. Ricketts. Ann Arbor: Health Administration Press.

Ottensmeyer, D. J. 1995. Proving value, aligning incentives, physician leadership, and creating a unified culture. Presentation at Integrated Healthcare Symposium, Aspen, Colo., 25–26 September.

Phillips, L. 1996. Lovelace Health Systems: A "living laboratory" for disease management. *Future fact: Demand management series*. Chicago: Hospital Research and Educational Trust.

Plainte, K. 1995. Developing an integrated delivery system for Medicare managed care. Presentation at Medicare Managed Care, Dallas, September.

Podbielski, J. 1996. Interview by author. Fallon Clinic, Inc., Worcester, Mass., 15 July.

Rainmakers: Allina moves the market. 1995. In *Pacesetters* (supplement to *Hospitals and Health Networks*). Chicago: American Hospital Publishing, Inc.

Reep, J. A. 1995. Who has the best information system for integrated health systems? Presentation at Integrated Healthcare Symposium, Aspen, Colo., 25–26 September.

Roberts, C. 1996. Interview by author. Copley Health System, Morrisville, Vt., 19 June and 12 August.

Rogers, M. C., R. Snyderman, and E. L. Rogers. 1994. Cultural and organizational implications of academic managed care networks. *New England Journal of Medicine* 331 (20): 1374–1377 (17 November).

Sandrick, K. 1995. If you want to play, you've got to pay. *Hospitals and Health Networks* 69 (13): 25–27 (5 July).

Schultz, D. V. 1995. The importance of primary care providers in integrated systems. *Healthcare Financial Management* 49: 58–63 (January).

Scott, K. 1997. Sentara Health System: Reinventing the organization. *Health System Leader* 4: 21–30 (March).

Shortell, S. M., R. R. Gillies, D. A. Anderson, K. M. Erickson, and J. B. Mitchell. 1996. *Remaking health care in America: Building organized delivery systems*. San Francisco: Jossey-Bass.

Southwick, K. 1995. Disease management broadens focus of care from episode to long-range. *Strategies for Healthcare Excellence* 8 (6): 1–5 (June).

————. 1996. Conservative care, "consumer government," and low premiums mean high-value care at Group Health Cooperative. *Strategies for Healthcare Excellence* 9 (4): 1–8 (April).

Stodghill, R. 1996. Attack of the health-care colossus. *Business Week* (20 May).

Telemedicine is a tool you can use to build your managed care network. 1996. *Hospital Managed Care Strategies* 4 (8): 85–88 (August).

Votz, D., and J. D. Cochrane. 1996. The future of provider-sponsored HMOs. *Integrated Healthcare Report* 1–8 (August).

White, S. 1997. Interview by author. Carolinas HealthCare System, Charlotte, N.C., 25 April.

Williams, C. 1996. CDM. *Appalachian Regional Healthcare Compendium* 6–9 (winter/spring).

Wittrup, R. D., V. K. Sahney, and G. L. Warden. 1994. Building a culture of participation in a vertically integrated, regional health system. In *Successful Strategies for Building an Integrated Hospital/Physician Healthcare System.* Rockville, Md.: Bader & Associates.

Yandell, L. 1997. Interview by author. Premier, Charlotte, N.C., 9 April.

Zablocki, E. 1996. Collaborating with competitors for healthier communities. *Health System Leader* 3 (10): 4–12 (December).

Zane, E. 1996. Interview by author. Partners HealthCare System, Inc., Boston, 18 April.

7

Case Study: Duke University Medical Center & Health System

INTRODUCTION

Duke University Medical Center (DUMC) in Durham, N.C., is one of the nation's premier academic medical centers. Rated fifth in the country in *US News and World Report's* ranking of best U.S. hospitals (Brink 1996) and often cited for its innovation, DUMC has long

---

Author's Note: The case study on Duke University Medical Center & Health System is based on my experience and the perceptions of many colleagues who worked there during 1992–1996—the years when Duke began to move beyond an academic medical center toward an integrated system. In my opinion, the most significant accomplishments of those early years were the strengthening of primary care capability, the willingness to assume financial risk for a defined population, and the transition of the faculty practice plan into a multispecialty group practice. As Duke moves forward in its growth as a system, however, it must address several difficult and sensitive issues. If the medical center expects to function as an integrated system, it must deal with system governance versus medical center governance. Furthermore, it must focus on long-range planning as a system. Creative and entrepreneurial visionaries who pass through North Carolina are no substitute for systemwide consensus on future direction. Finally, Duke must deal with its responsibility in creating healthier communities.

enjoyed a reputation for excellence in education, research, and clinical practice.

In the early 1990s, Duke faced the same threats as other academic medical centers. The health care market was moving rapidly toward managed care. Duke's insistence on higher prices for better quality fell on deaf ears, as managed care plans refused to pay for the high cost of education and research that affected all academic medical centers. Decreases in clinical revenue changed the balance between clinical and academic dollars, forcing the medical center to reduce costs and seek new sources of support. Internally, organizational structures that remained unchanged for many years obstructed the organization from meeting new planning and operational challenges on a timely basis. Fewer trainees were needed, and the curriculum needed modernization.

Writing in the *New England Journal of Medicine* in late 1994, medical center leaders were direct about their dilemma: "The real threat that managed care poses to the academic medical center is financial insolvency" (Rogers, Snyderman, and Rogers 1994). With this thought in mind, Duke embarked upon a multiphase development of an integrated delivery system—the Duke University Medical Center & Health System—that would build on core missions and existing strengths and make the medical center more competitive in a changing environment.

Accomplishments during the first phase of Duke's development of an integrated system included the following:

- Strengthening primary care capability
- Preliminary development of a continuum of care
- Selective partnering with a major insurance company and a major supplier
- Assumption of full financial risk for a defined population
- Transition of the faculty practice plan into a more efficiently run multispecialty group practice
- Achievement of major cost reductions
- Evaluation of information systems
- Development of case/care management

All those accomplishments reflected Duke's commitment to teaching, research, and clinical practice. Advantages that Duke brought to the challenge were a robust organization, vision and motivation, talent, experience in solutions through science, and an educational focus (Snyderman 1996).

This case study of the Duke University Medical Center & Health System is divided into the following sections:

- Background
- Special issues facing academic medical centers
- Phase I accomplishments
- Barriers
- Future challenges

BACKGROUND

Description of Duke University Medical Center

Prior to the 1990s, DUMC's structure (fig. 7-1) resembled that of many academic medical centers. Medical center components included Duke Hospital, the School of Medicine, the School of Nursing, Allied Health, Graduate Medical Education, and the faculty practice plan (private diagnostic clinic, or PDC).

FIGURE 7-1. Traditional Organization Chart of Duke University Medical Center

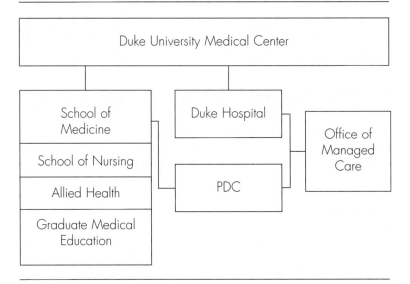

Clinical operations were centered in Duke Hospital and the PDC. By 1995, Duke Hospital had become one of the largest teaching hospitals in the country. Its annual volume of inpatient admissions was 36,000, and the volume of outpatient visits exceeded 500,000. Duke excelled in tertiary and specialty care. The PDC was a limited liability partnership affiliated with Duke University. Like most faculty practice plans, it was dominated by specialists.

Although Duke Hospital and the PDC were separate legal entities, the Medical Center Office of Managed Care, which was founded in the early 1990s, coordinated managed care contracting for both. Initially, DUMC resisted managed care. When failure to price competitively resulted in the potential loss of a large block of business, the contracting strategy changed to aggressive pricing and accommodation to market demands. Although many of Duke's early agreements had been for specialty care, Duke's portfolio of contracts began to expand beyond specialty areas like the heart center and transplant programs that had been particularly responsive to managed care needs. Many of the newer contracts were full-service agreements and direct employer contracts.

DUMC patients came from three service areas: local, immediate, and outlying. The local service area was defined as Durham, Orange, and Wake counties. The immediate service area included other counties within an hour's drive from the medical center. Finally, the outlying service area included all other counties in North Carolina, other states, and foreign countries. Patients' willingness to drive up to four hours to Durham made the rural market very important; many people from distant communities bypassed other academic medical centers closer to their homes to go to Duke.

North Carolina Health Care Environment

Compared with other regions of the country, managed care came late to North Carolina. DUMC thus had an opportunity to learn from the experiences of medical centers in other states. In 1992, an estimated 6 to 7 percent of residents in the state were enrolled in managed care. Penetration varied significantly depending on urban and rural locations. In urban areas like the Raleigh/Durham/Chapel Hill Triangle, penetration was 13 to 14 percent. In rural areas, many of which had an undersupply of primary care caregivers, penetration was low. At DUMC, only 3 percent of 1993 discharges were managed care enrollees.

These statistics were misleading when one looked at the kind of health plan classified as "managed." For the most part, managed care meant enrollment in PPOs that lacked strong primary care physician management and provider financial risk. Even in HMO plans, the concept of enrollee management by primary care physicians who act as gatekeepers was uncommon; many North Carolina HMOs prided themselves on their ability to survive without primary care management.

In the public sector, the North Carolina Department of Human Resources, Division of Medical Assistance (DMA) had developed Carolina Access, a primary care physician model program. The program was mandatory for Medicaid recipients in six categories in those counties with the capacity to provide service and interest in participation. Enrollees selected a primary care physician who was expected to coordinate all other care. Physicians were paid according to a Medicaid fee schedule, and primary care physicians received a small administrative fee to manage the care of enrollees who selected them. There were no strong incentives to either providers or enrollees to abide by program rules.

By 1996, with the threat of federal changes looming, the DMA planned to introduce mandatory capitated managed care in one North Carolina county and to expand that model in other urban areas. Simultaneously, 12 providers across the state, including DUMC, were developing an alternative provider-driven Medicaid managed care option.

Medicare managed care was in its infancy. Kaiser had developed a small cost-based program for enrollees age 65 and older. Most of the other managed care plans were concentrating on the commercial market and were not planning managed care for seniors.

North Carolina was a state where managed care was waiting to happen; DUMC recognized that opportunity.

SPECIAL ISSUES FACING ACADEMIC MEDICAL CENTERS

At the time DUMC decided to develop the Duke University Medical Center & Health System, it faced many of the problems unique to academic medical centers, including the following:

- Historic balance between clinical practice and research
- High cost of care relative to that offered by nonacademic providers
- Payer mix that included both managed and nonmanaged care
- Challenge of teaching attending physicians, residents, and medical students about practicing in a managed care environment
- Difficulty of using an academic medical center structure for decision making in a managed care environment
- Impact of relationship with the university of which it is a part
- Conflict between the historic focus on tertiary/specialty care and managed care's emphasis on primary care

Balance between Clinical Practice and Research

Historically, DUMC's research efforts had been supported by multiple sources: clinical revenues, government, industry, and not-for-profit private foundations. The reduction in clinical revenues caused by changes in health insurance created pressure to increase research support from all nonclinical areas. Duke responded by creating the Office of Science and Technology (OST) and the Duke Clinical Research Institute (CRI).

The universitywide OST was established to enhance Duke's ability to increase nonclinical support. Its head reported directly to the chancellor for health affairs/dean of the school of medicine. As expected, the development of partnerships with industry improved faculty recruitment, funding for new research, and enhancement of core technologies (Snyderman 1995).

The Duke CRI was created to improve quantitative information and allow better medical practice. Priorities were collaborative clinical investigation and partnerships among centers that could collectively improve the performance and dissemination of research. In creating the CRI, Duke expanded its strong cardiovascular research foundation to include multiple clinical disciplines.

Cost of Care

In the early 1990s, the cost of care at DUMC was high compared with that of nonacademic institutions. In fact, even after Duke's commitment to managed care, the cost of care in the Triangle geographic area compared unfavorably with that in other urban areas (Harreld 1996). Managed care health plans would not support those high costs, and Duke's contract pricing strategy changed.

Negotiating more competitive contracts was just the first step; the more difficult challenge was reduction in the cost of delivering care. Duke Hospital had shown a healthy cumulative surplus of $70 million to $75 million in 1991 and 1992. By 1993, the size of the surplus had dropped, and without major cost reduction efforts, the hospital faced a deficit. Both Duke Hospital and the PDC undertook a number of initiatives, several of which contained joint financial incentives for both hospital and physicians. These initiatives included the following:

- A two-year effort to reduce hospital costs by $70 million and eliminate 1,500 positions with minimum layoffs
- A joint venture with a major supplier that created incentives for both provider and supplier
- A program to share a portion of hospital savings with physicians

Payer Mix

Although medical center leaders anticipated a dramatic shift in payer mix, in the early 1990s, most of Duke's patients, including Duke University employees, were covered by commercial insurance. The only identifiable group with "managed care" insurance were 2,000 Medicaid clients enrolled in Carolina Access. As has already been mentioned, that program lacked the essential ingredient for managed care—provider financial risk.

A payer mix dominated by managed care was not yet a reality. Neither patients from rural areas nor international patients had managed care insurance. Because many of the international and commercially insured patients paid full charges for care, much of the medical center lacked the incentive to change.

Duke University's decision to change the health insurance for 34,000 employees and dependents became the catalyst for change. The Duke employees were a visible and vocal group. When health insurance options and procedures for accessing care changed for them, the message of managed care hit home.

Teaching Challenges

The concepts and practices of managed care needed to be taught to four audiences. Both faculty and private physicians needed to understand new expectations. Their office staff needed to understand new kinds of health insurance and related administrative requirements. Hospital administrative and clinical staff needed similar education. Finally, medical students and residents needed to understand the environment in which they were likely to practice medicine and its implications for clinical care. All four audiences needed to learn that "good" care extended beyond clinical excellence and included patient/enrollee concerns: access to care, shortened waiting times, smooth referral processes, physician understanding, adherence to authorization and certification requirements, and improved communication between physicians themselves and between physicians and patients.

With respect to physicians, managed care was initially explained in a "hands on" rather than a philosophical manner. The shift of Duke University employees and dependents into Duke Managed Care in July 1995 prompted many questions about clinical and administrative systems by both enrollees and the health plan. For example, Duke clinicians were surprised to learn that "medical necessity" in health plan terms had a meaning different from what they had expected.

Several newly created groups assumed leadership roles in conveying the importance of managed care to practicing physicians, including the following:

- Joint Venture Managed Care Operations Committee: Formed to facilitate the operational aspects of Duke Managed Care, this committee represented Duke Health Network and NYLCare (co-chairs), Duke Hospital, the PDC, and Duke University Affiliated Physicians (DUAP).
- PDC Managed Care Committee: One of four PDC standing committees, this group provided overall guidance on managed care policy issues, including but not limited to Duke Managed Care.
- PDC Managed Care Committee/Physicians: Accountable to the PDC Managed Care Committee, this group represented most specialties and DUAP. It dealt with operational issues such as practice guidelines, disease management, physician profiling, and day-to-day practice management.

- PDC Primary Care Committee: Representing both the faculty practice and DUAP physicians, this group was instrumental in redefining the relationships of primary care and specialist physicians and in clarifying the role of primary care physicians in managing patient care.

With respect to educating physicians' office staff, the challenge for both the PDC and DUAP was to centralize and standardize activities that had historically been decentralized. The office and clinical staff of Duke faculty physicians included employees paid by the hospital, PDC, and individual physician. In any given location, then, there were employees with three sets of priorities. The DUAP office staff were accustomed to receiving instructions from individual physicians, not from a centralized administration in a large academic medical practice.

At Duke Hospital, teaching managed care occurred in two ways. As with the physicians, the conversion to Duke Managed Care required changes for everyone and accelerated the learning process. Also, and equally important, Duke signed a variety of managed care contracts that required provider assumption of financial risk. For each new risk contract, contracting staff worked with hospital staff to explain the plan-specific requirements and solve operational problems.

Finally, and very important, Duke formalized changes in the medical school curriculum late in 1995. Highlights (Bhatt 1995; Snyderman 1995) of those changes include the following:

- Definition of a contemporary core curriculum
- Problem-based learning
- Continuity of care curriculum in integrating ambulatory setting, health prevention, and education
- Mandatory clerkship in cost-effectiveness
- Community-based learning, including a requirement for all fourth-year students to spend at least four weeks in an ambulatory setting
- Increased emphasis on primary care
- Master's in Public Health and Clinical Epidemiology as an alternative to basic research for third-year students

Decision-Making Structure

Although DUMC took a bold step in developing a health system, its structure did not change at the same speed as its long-term goals.

DUMC leaders themselves recognized this inconsistency (Rogers, Snyderman, and Rogers 1994). Among Duke's problems were lack of hierarchy, customary functioning in small groups rather than teams or systems, and departmental autonomy.

The structure at Duke reflected that of a typical not-for-profit academic medical center. In contrast to the for-profit sector, lines of responsibility were not always clear. Financial support came from multiple sources, fostering the notion of independence. Individuals, departments, and divisions took great pride in their entrepreneurial spirit and accomplishments.

Another structural problem was the relationship between DUMC and Duke University trustees. Historically, the university's full board and executive committee had devoted a considerable amount of time and attention to medical center affairs. The DUMC trustee committee of the board had been involved in some of the confidentiality issues such as litigation and credentialing. Both the university board and medical center leadership realized that this structure often handicapped full understanding of issues and delayed decision making in a rapidly changing environment.

Four changes facilitated DUMC's ability to function in a competitive market:

- Creation of a new standing university board committee, the Trustee Committee for the Duke University Health System
- Creation of a new decision-making body, the Clinical Operations Committee
- Creation of the Duke Health Network to take charge of entrepreneurial efforts during system start-up
- Changes in PDC governance and operations

The new standing committee of the university board, the Trustee Committee for the Duke University Health System, was formed to devote full attention to the affairs of the Duke Health System. Elected by the board, the committee comprised a minimum of 13 members, the majority of whom were trustees. Nontrustee members included knowledgeable health care and business professionals.

The Clinical Operations Committee was created to act as the "board" of the Duke Health System (Snyderman 1995). It included the chancellor for health affairs, the medical center CFO, the Duke Hospital CEO and COO, the Duke Health Network COO, and PDC physicians. The committee offered its members an opportunity to share information and financial details with a new openness.

The Duke Health Network was created to handle the initial entrepreneurial challenges of building a system (fig. 7-2). Both Duke Hospital and the PDC faculty practice plan provided financial support. Network activities did not fit into the traditional medical center structure and were best organized separately. These included physician practice acquisition, development of a joint venture with an insurance company, managed care contracting and operations, physician consultation and referral services, affiliations (outreach) with physicians and hospitals in more than 30 communities, analytic support for both the hospital and physicians, and planning for public sector managed care programs.

The PDC faculty practice plan made major organizational changes to address the managed care environment (fig. 7-3). The governance structure included a single PDC administrative board and four standing committees: PDC affairs, managed care, primary care, and clinical affairs. Functions that had previously been departmentally run, such as appointments, scheduling, billing, and communications, were centralized. Although the en masse conversion of Duke University employees and dependents to managed care was difficult, the PDC administrative changes made the process easier than it otherwise would have been.

Relationship with the University of Which It Is Part

DUMC is a part of a larger university. Duke University, not DUMC, changed the health insurance of 34,000 employees and dependents. Duke University human resources revised the benefit package, the cost-sharing arrangements, and other parameters. This important distinction between university and medical center was frequently lost on employees, especially physicians and contentious faculty members of the general academic campus.

For example, six months after the change in employee health insurance, faculty and staff continued to vocalize concerns about the university's decision (Arnold 1995). Complaints centered around the small number of available insurance options (two) and the "quality" of the Duke Managed Care option. Another aspect of the new insurance that resulted in public employee objection was the coverage for developmental disabilities.

Freedom of thought and expression is characteristic of an academic environment. Neither Duke University nor the medical center expected to stifle criticism. An independent audit of Duke

FIGURE 7-2. Duke Health Network Organization Chart (1992–1996)

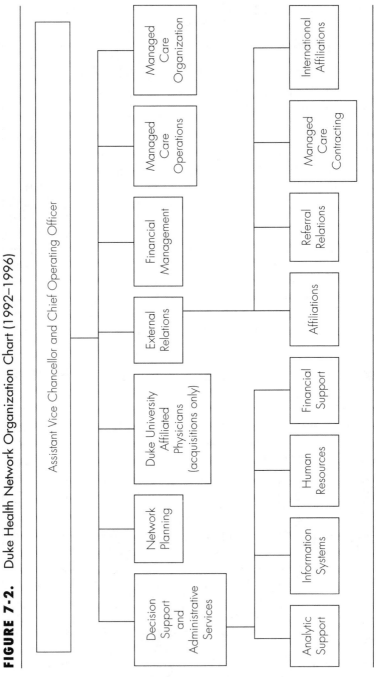

FIGURE 7-3. New PDC Committees (1994)

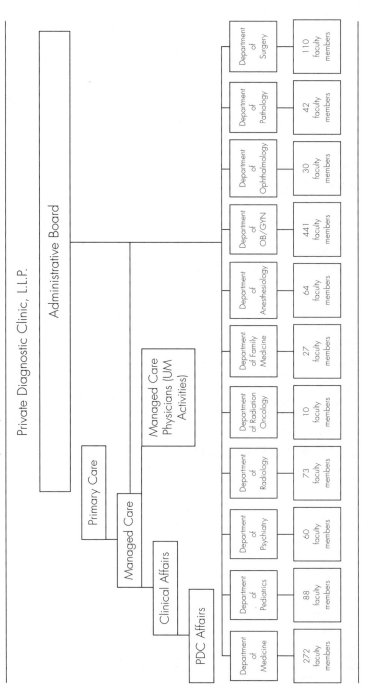

Managed Care by A. Foster Higgins & Co. was commissioned by the university to determine if the health plan was structured in a way that ensured it was operating in the best interests of its members. The results were favorable to the plan. In a statement issued one year after the change in health insurance, university human resources indicated that the financial savings had been significant (Zimmer 1996).

Conflict between Emphases on Tertiary/ Specialty Care and Primary Care

Historically, Duke excelled in tertiary and specialty care. The faculty practice plan included primary care physicians in internal medicine and pediatrics. However, prior to July 1995, the entire division of community and family medicine was not part of the PDC partnership.

Recognizing the importance of primary care in a managed care environment, DUMC took three important steps to strengthen it. First, it created DUAP, a separate corporation empowered to acquire community primary care physicians. Second, the division of family medicine became part of the PDC partnership. Third, the PDC created a primary care standing committee and began the administrative and geographic consolidation of its separate practices.

ACCOMPLISHMENTS

During the 1992–1996 initial phase of the development of its health system, Duke accomplished the following:

- Strengthened primary care throughout the local/immediate service area
- Began development of a continuum of care to include enhanced ambulatory services and alternative sites
- Selectively partnered with a major insurance company and a major supplier in joint risk arrangements
- Assumed full financial risk for a population of 34,000 Duke University employees and dependents
- Transitioned the faculty practice plan into a more efficient multispecialty group practice

- Achieved major cost reductions
- Evaluated appropriateness of existing information systems
- Developed case/care management

Strengthened Primary Care

Primary care capability has a direct impact on an integrated system's ability to attract and manage the health and wellness of discrete populations. Duke's primary care capacity was inadequate for a target population of 850,000. Access to primary care was another problem; geographically, all primary care was provided at the medical center and at several nearby sites. However, those locations were not convenient to the growing population moving into outlying areas.

To enhance primary care, Duke acquired 56 physicians in 18 practice sites. Community and family medicine physician faculty were integrated into the PDC partnership. In 1996 the PDC made a decision to hire a single primary care medical director and administrator. A new primary care site for physicians in general internal medicine, general pediatrics, and community and family medicine opened in July 1996. By 1997, the Medical Outpatient Clinic was relocated to a site that would improve patient access, teaching, and the delivery of patient care.

Developed Continuum of Care

Historically, Duke's strength and reputation had been earned in the provision of inpatient acute, tertiary, and quaternary care. To attract managed care plans and enrollees, Duke's new system needed a broader scope of services that included prevention and wellness, enhanced ambulatory care, home care, long-term care, and other alternatives to hospitalization.

With respect to health prevention and wellness, the medical center had many ongoing but unconnected initiatives. In summer 1995, internal inventories revealed a large number of uncoordinated formal and informal efforts. The more well-known programs included Duke Diet & Fitness Program, the Live for Life program for employees, and the Duke Center for Living. Different clinical areas took pride in their homegrown prevention and education programs. Once the inventories were completed, Duke began the consolidation process.

The initial Duke strategy for home care, long-term care, and other alternative types of care was to develop collaborative relationships. An example was a partnership with Boston-based Chartwell Home Therapies and the creation of Chartwell Southeast. Initially, DUMC did not believe it needed to own all aspects of the continuum.

Began Selective Partnering

A major component of DUMC's managed care strategy was selective partnering with for-profit companies in relationships that included shared financial risk for both partners. Important partnership relationships were developed with NYLCare (formerly New York Life/Sanus), Baxter Healthcare Corporation, Hewlett-Packard, and Johnson & Johnson.

DUMC and NYLCare created a joint venture to offer a commercial insurance product throughout North Carolina. WellPath Community Health Plans Holding, LLC, was licensed in late 1995 to operate as an HMO in 44 counties. NYLCare and Duke also collaborated in developing Duke Managed Care, a self-insured POS product for Duke University employees (N.Y. Life 1995). The partnership with NYLCare was a jump-start for Duke, taking it quickly into the capitated managed care arena.

With respect to Baxter Healthcare Corporation, the world's largest hospital supply company, Duke signed a five-year managed cost agreement that aligned the financial incentives of both organizations around reducing total system costs. Standardization, utilization, and process improvements occurred. The mutually favorable results of the Duke/Baxter project encouraged DUMC to seek out other mutually beneficial relationships with industry.

Assumed Full Financial Risk for a Large Population

On July 1, 1995, Duke University's new health insurance plan took effect. Almost all of the 34,000 employees and dependents moved into the Duke Managed Care plan, a POS option. The plan was self-insured by Duke University. NYLCare of North Carolina was the third-party administrator.

The financial terms of the agreement between NYLCare and DUMC put both Duke Hospital and physicians at risk. All physicians—

primary care and specialist, PDC, and DUAP—shared that risk. The financial arrangements put the entire Duke provider community on the same playing field, giving everyone parallel financial incentives.

Duke's commitment to accept full financial risk was a bold step. Prior to the initiation of Duke Managed Care, Duke Hospital and the PDC physicians had negotiated managed care contracts with minor risk provisions, but none of those agreements had required so large a commitment. Although the infrastructure to manage under risk arrangements was in its infancy, intellectually the medical center believed that acceptance of risk under capitation was the appropriate approach given its long-term plans.

Transitioned the Faculty Practice Plan into a Multispecialty Group Practice

The PDC, Duke's faculty practice plan of 800 physicians, made a number of changes in governance, administration, and operations to adapt to a managed care environment and assume a leadership role in the development of an integrated system.

PDC governance was changed to reflect the priorities that the entire partnership needed to face. Three of the four standing committees (managed care, primary care, and clinical affairs) dealt regularly with the issues of managed care. Administratively, the PDC centralized many of the functions that had previously been done by divisions and departments. The partnership was converted to a limited liability corporation. Finally, the PDC created a management services organization to facilitate its relationships with other physicians in other communities.

Achieved Major Cost Reductions

DUMC undertook major cost reduction efforts at the same time that it engaged in system-building activities. The first component of cost reduction, operations improvement, was designed to restructure hospital operations. Stanford and Vanderbilt Medical Centers were the models. Not only did these improvements take $70 million dollars out of a $550 million operating budget; they also changed the way people worked. Two other successful cost reduction strategies for Duke Hospital addressed capital equipment and product standardization.

Evaluated Existing Information Systems

In 1991, DUMC management realized that the information systems that supported administrative and clinical operations were not sufficient to meet the future demands of the Duke University Medical Center & Health System. Duke's existing systems included the following elements:

- Duke Hospital Information Systems (DHIS) for patient accounting and billing, laboratory, pharmacy, radiology, and other services
- IDX for support of clinic administrative functions (for example, appointment scheduling and billing)
- Isolated systems developed internally by clinical departments to support clinical research (for example, cardiovascular database)
- T1, a decision support product from Transition Systems, Inc.

Although most of these systems produced virtually flawless transaction processing work, they were unable to fulfill the growing needs of a health system. Like most mainframe-based legacy systems, DHIS did not lend itself to changes and enhancements; modifications were labor intensive, time consuming, and expensive. Because DHIS and IDX shared only patient demographic information, inpatient and outpatient data were not integrated. Limited clinical information such as diagnosis and procedure codes were integrated with financial and administrative information. Department-specific clinical information systems did not permit cross-department integration, although many Duke patients received care from clinicians in different disciplines. Finally, because mainframe-based DHIS and its constellation of dumb terminals provided most of the automated support for both hospital and clinic functions, Duke could not take full advantage of technological advances.

Recognizing the limitations of its existing information systems, Duke conducted a search for a new hospital information system to replace DHIS. Following months of proposal review, demonstrations from various vendors, and site visits to other academic medical centers, it was determined that no one system on the market at the time would meet Duke's needs. Furthermore, what DHIS did, it did well; it simply was unable to provide the new functionality required in a world where managed care would dominate.

With the recruitment and hiring of a new chief information officer, Duke altered its information systems/information technology (IS/IT) path and developed a different strategy. Its essence was to revamp Duke's information system infrastructure design so that Duke was better positioned to respond to internal demands for information and take advantage of developing new technologies. The new IS/IT strategy had the following components:

- Refocus of IS/IT project management to accommodate strategic as well as operational projects
- Selective "deconstruction" of DHIS, including installation of 20 department systems with more than 70 HL7 interfaces, installation of a message router to facilitate information exchange, and creation of a common data respository (CDR) to facilitate integration of administrative, financial, and clinical information and improve clinician access to clinical data
- Emphasis on personal computers (PCs) rather than terminals, and development of PC-based applications to meet institutional needs for uniformity and consistency while recognizing unique department needs (for example, browser and inbox)
- Recognition of the entrepreneurial nature of Duke's culture so that medical center IS/IT strategic planning supports, not stifles, creativity

The change in Duke's IS/IT strategy had three important results. First, the medical center's "systems agility" philosophy has allowed the institution to take full advantage of evolving new technologies. Second, clinicians are supportive of the changes because they now have greater access to clinical information. Third, Duke now has a technical architectural infrastructure which allows the IS department to respond to new business initiatives with an information component. An example is DUAP, the primary care physicians that Duke purchased as part of system development.

Developed Case/Care Management

Most of DUMC's initial system-building efforts were directed toward putting the components of a system in place. Early on, however, it became very clear that Duke needed to improve the way it managed the patients who received care. The loss of a major managed care contract to a competitor was the catalyst that inspired the development of case management. The initial program was just a start in what was expected to evolve into a systemwide effort.

Case/care management began at Duke in 1995. All inpatients were screened according to specific criteria and categorized as needing one of five levels of case management. The first-year goal was to hire 22 specialty-specific case managers, each of whom would have responsibility for all inpatients in particular units regardless of payer class.

Although inpatient case management was the priority, there was an immediate need for a case manager to handle the large group of university employees and dependents who had moved into managed care; consequently, a Duke Managed Care case manager was put in place. Other groups as well, such as enrollees in another risk plan, needed special attention. With respect to ambulatory case management, the physicians were not yet comfortable with the idea. Rather than unveil a broad and expensive program, Duke began with a "hot line" ambulatory case manager accessible to all primary care physicians who felt he or she had a particularly complex patient to manage and wanted to use the resource.

BARRIERS

During the initial development of its health system, DUMC encountered at least eight barriers, including the following:

- Difficulty in clarifying system missions, goals, and strategies
- Downsizing an acute hospital
- Gluing components together to create patient-focused processes of care
- Moving beyond contracting into operations
- Juggling joint venture equity partnership with other managed care relationships
- Understanding the role of research in managed care
- Addressing cultural obstacles
- Emphasizing market-driven mentality rather than delivery system capabilities

Difficulty in Clarifying System Mission, Goals, and Strategies

During the initial phase, responsibility for developing and implementing the Duke University Medical Center & Health System was lodged within the traditional medical center structure. The new clinical operations committee and the Duke Health Network were important new entities, but both were creatures of the medical center. Neither clearly articulated the health system mission, goals, and strategy in ways that adequately addressed internal and external confusion about the new direction that the medical center was taking.

Downsizing

To DUMC leadership, it was inevitable that the size of Duke Hospital would decrease from 1,000 in the early 1990s to a level of approximately 750 beds. To practicing physicians, the reduction of inpatient capacity was not yet a reality. In fact, the threat of downsizing inpatient capacity motivated several specialty areas to explore ways to establish ambulatory "outposts" that might feed volume back to Duke Hospital and compensate for lost inpatient business.

Over time, faculty physicians focused less on generating inpatient volume than they did on improving the efficiency of the delivery of care. For example, surgeons specializing in breast surgery shortened hospital stay, reduced patient discomfort, and improved the quality of care by changing the type of anesthesia used. The need to manage so many Duke University employees was an important catalyst.

Moving beyond Contracting into Operations

As a novice in managed care, neither Duke Hospital nor Duke's physicians had experience in changing operations to accommodate managed care. To most people, managed care implied contract negotiations—that is, how many contracts and at what reimbursement level. Less attention was devoted to what would happen after these contracts were signed.

Duke University's venture into managed care under a capitated arrangement challenged the entire delivery system. Administrative, clinical, and communication problems quickly surfaced. Two examples were the sharing of information and the implementation of the POS option.

With respect to information, when specialists recommended a procedure or surgery, their offices generally scheduled whatever needed to be done. Information was not routinely communicated to the primary care physician or to the health plan. Often, the proverbial cart moved ahead of the horse, and patients were scheduled for treatment or surgery before appropriate approvals were obtained. Once patient expectations had been set, administrative staff were uncomfortable causing delays to conform to health plan requirements.

The implementation of the Duke Managed Care POS option created another operational problem. The POS concept was new for Duke; most managed care plans in North Carolina offered an HMO or PPO. When the plan started, Duke Managed Care enrollees who appeared in specialist offices without appropriate primary care physician authorization received care. Administrative staff sought retroactive approval under the assumption that they were being patient-friendly. In fact, the process undermined the goal of the POS benefit—that is, to encourage enrollees to seek in-network care with proper authorization/approval.

Gluing Components Together to Create Patient-Focused Processes of Care

At DUMC, as at most academic medical centers, the organizational structure was not "lean and mean." Duke Hospital and the PDC partnership had separate structures and budgets, and department chairs also controlled portions of funding. Although there was cross-subsidization among the different entities, it was difficult to convince the separate "silos" to work together on common problem solving. Coordination of important systems functions was difficult, as illustrated by information systems and case/care management.

Information systems at DUMC had both information and people problems. The medical center had multiple information systems but no patient-focused computerized medical record linking clinical and financial information together. Duke Hospital and the faculty practice plan had different systems. Although they ultimately linked their cost accounting systems, clinical information remained separate. Other separate systems contained laboratory and pharmacy information. Furthermore, the primary care practices that Duke purchased were not linked to each other or to the medical center, and it was difficult to report test results back to these physicians.

To improve its future direction, Duke and IBM collaborated in the HealthLink project. Its goal was to create for the Duke University Medical Center & Health System health data networks that would provide payers, employers, and health care organizations the information they needed to manage patient care across the continuum.

Another problem with information systems related to people. Although physicians and other caregivers intellectually supported the idea of using clinical and financial information to monitor their practices and improve the delivery of care, it was unclear who would use that information to effect change. Practice guidelines, physician profiling, and case management information systems were in the making, but there was ambiguity regarding responsibility to use it.

The development of care management also presented a challenge in coordination. Duke Hospital had placed case management within the division of patient services. Physicians in the faculty practice plan and newly acquired practices had been involved in the adaptation of external practice guidelines to meet Duke needs. A physician committee had been charged with the responsibility for utilization management, but the ways in which all these activities would come together were still unclear.

Juggling Joint Venture Equity Partnership with Other Managed Care Relationships

Duke's decision to create a joint venture with NYLCare was a major one. Although university employees represented only 8 percent of hospital inpatient volume, the visibility of the change and the fact that physicians and staff would personally be affected increased the impact of the decision.

The process for selecting an insurance partner was competitive and resulted in the selection of a major national carrier. The immediate reaction of those plans not selected was that they did not want to do business with DUMC. Over time, some of those plans realized that Duke's decision to commit to managed care and to accept risk under capitated payments would benefit them; these plans continued to deal with Duke.

Within Duke, however, it took time to sort out the meaning of the joint venture insurance partnership. Did it mean that in all efforts, the joint venture partner received priority treatment, or did it mean that the partnership was important and that other opportunities were to be pursued as well? Ultimately, Duke decided that the joint venture partnership would not replace all other contracts, and that the medical center needed to develop and maintain many relationships.

Understanding the Role of Research in Managed Care

The role of research in managed care was a thorny one for DUMC, as it is for all academic medical centers. Research represented nearly one-fourth of the entire $950 million institutional budget.

Shortly after the ink was dry on the Duke joint venture with NYLCare, the issue of insurer reimbursement for clinical trials surfaced. The medical center launched a study to determine the impact of managed care on all clinical trials.

A positive way in which Duke related research to managed care was in disease management. Information on Duke's own employees/families and on other groups of patients indicated that certain categories of patients accounted for a large proportion of the health care dollar. Toward the end of the first phase of system development, Duke identified those high-cost diseases and initiated an effort to develop a model approach to multidisciplinary disease management.

Addressing Cultural Obstacles

The cultural barriers to change in an academic medical center were well understood by its leaders (Rogers, Snyderman, and Rogers 1994). These constraints included but were not limited to the following:

- Respect for freedom to question
- Division of faculty time among administration, clinical care, and research

- Unclear clinical and administrative expectations
- Ambiguity of medical faculty, administration, and hospital roles
- Resistance to external ideas and pride in homegrown solutions
- Devotion to development of consensus
- Reliance on traditional medical center structures to make new decisions
- Emphasis on individualism versus collaboration
- Clinician rather than patient focus

DUMC's approach to all the cultural obstacles was to accept them as constraints and move onward.

Emphasizing Market-Driven Mentality

As a medical center renowned for specialty care, DUMC suffered from an attitude common at academic medical centers: "If we organize, provide, and price care the way we want to, patients will come." In a managed care environment, however, patients do not always come, and their insurance does not always pay. Although "carve-out" strategies for cardiovascular care, transplants, and mental health/substance abuse were appropriate to payer needs, carving out other subspecialty areas was less attractive. Over time, Duke clinicians began to get the message—that payers and enrollees did not want fragmented and uncoordinated care. They wanted coordination of care by primary care and specialist physicians supported by case/care management.

FUTURE CHALLENGES

Like many developing integrated systems, DUMC made a quick exit from the starting gate. Its early accomplishments were made within a relatively short time frame. Medical center leadership took an aggressive approach, and physicians and administration were willing to try a variety of new approaches. Nonetheless, "systems don't just happen" (Shortell and others 1996).

During the next phase of system development, DUMC will reevaluate the marketplace. One external factor has remained constant: clinical revenues will continue to decrease. In other respects, however, the scenario is very different from 1992. First, two large populations important to Duke (Medicaid and Medicare) are likely to move into managed care. Second, large for-profit hospital systems are expanding their North Carolina presence. Third, large national physician-owned companies are competing for physicians. Fourth, health plans and insurers are likely to consolidate as new large national players move into the North Carolina market.

In this new environment, Duke must address the following:

- System vision and organization
- System responsibility for the health and wellness of discrete populations
- Application of research techniques and findings to specific groups of patients and populations
- Appropriate delivery system structure for the provision of care and services
- Expansion of preliminary efforts in IS/IT and care management

System Vision and Organization

Although Duke's accomplishments during the first four years of systems development are impressive, two essential steps did not occur. Unless they do, its future as a system is uncertain. First, activities related to building an integrated system were performed, but without a formal planning process and agreement on system vision, goals, and objectives. Second, Duke did not address the appropriateness of the organizational structure of an academic medical center for an integrated health care system.

With respect to the lack of planning and agreement on a vision for the Duke System, Robert W. Anderson, MD, chairman of surgery and the managed care committee, described the problem in the initial session of the Duke Managed Care Education Program presented for Duke physicians. He suggested that change for the sake of change is no substitute for clarity of purpose and clear direction (Anderson 1996).

Four years into its system development, Duke remained organized like a traditional academic medical center. The faculty practice plan, the primary care physicians whom Duke had purchased,

Duke Hospital, and medical center administration were separate entities. Their priorities were different, and they competed for influence. Operational issues that spanned multiple organizations were difficult to resolve. Although people talked about a continuum of care and population-based planning, the organization structure remained a major obstacle to progress.

System Responsibility for the Health and Wellness of Discrete Populations

Many integrated systems identify as a major goal the assumption of responsibility for the health and wellness of discrete populations. Those populations may be enrollees in a system-owned health plan, payer-specific groups such as Medicaid and Medicare, or the community at large. Although the Duke University Medical Center & Health System did not identify population-based care as an organizational priority, many separate projects began to move in that direction.

Duke University's decision to change the health insurance of university employees and dependents to managed care, and the medical center's willingness to accept financial risk for that population, very quickly created an opportunity for the provider component of the Duke system to manage the health and wellness of Duke employees and their families. A pilot program in community and family medicine may be expanded to a larger base. The expectation that Medicaid and Medicare patients will soon be covered by managed care is expected to accelerate Duke's attention to population-based care. Finally, Duke University, including the medical center, has embarked on a major project to work more closely with neighborhoods adjacent to it.

Application of Research Techniques and Findings to Specific Populations

Toward the end of the first phase of its system development, Duke embarked on a disease management initiative. Asthma management by a multidisciplinary team of caregivers was used to test the concept. As Duke's program takes shape, it will have an important impact on the way in which care is delivered to specific populations and ultimately to all patients who go to Duke.

Delivery System Structure for Providing Care and Services

The Duke University Medical Center & Health System delivery system looks very different today from the way it looked in 1992. Most important is the strength of primary care. Efforts within the PDC and in DUAP have changed the traditional specialty-dominated balance in a way that is suitable for a managed care environment.

Other pieces of the continuum of care are less well developed. For example, at the outset, the Duke mind-set toward alternative nonacute care was that contractual relationships would suffice. That thinking has changed, and efforts are now under way to increase the number and type of ownership arrangements.

Another aspect of the delivery system that DUMC must address is the relationship between its own physicians and those in the many communities with which it has affiliations. Throughout North Carolina, hospital mergers and physician acquisitions have increased. As competition continues to grow, it will be necessary to formalize relationships that have been "gentlemen's agreements" for years. At the end of 1996, DUMC was exploring two options that are not mutually exclusive. One would add community physicians into the PDC; the other is the development of an IPA that would include Duke faculty, acquired physicians in DUAP, and community physicians.

Expansion of Preliminary Efforts in IS/IT and Care Management

Two of the most important parts of system infrastructure, IS/IT and care management, will be priorities for the Duke system in the future. With respect to IS/IT, at least five challenges lie ahead:

- The medical center should reevaluate its methodology for making capital allocation decisions for IS equipment so that IS/IT investment priorities are consistent with business strategies. An example is the balance between inpatient and outpatient systems.
- Greater focus should be given to decision support and exploitation of evolving information technologies. Examples are data mining and data warehousing.
- The IS/IT department organizational structure should support the evolving business structure and emphasize the

entire enterprise rather than separate hospital and clinical activities.

■ Information needs should be balanced with information system needs.

■ Duke's ability to respond to referring clinicians and outside health plans will depend on methodologies and strategies for sharing information with non-Duke clinicians.

With respect to care management, Duke must address the following issues:

■ Expansion of the scope of responsibility of care management beyond the inpatient focus and across the continuum of care

■ Improved collaboration between all members of the health care team

■ Development of a medical center utilization management program

Acknowledgments

The following individuals have provided input to the Duke case study:

Robert W. Anderson, MD
Janis Curtis
William J. Donelan
J. Lloyd Michener, MD
James J. Morris, MD
Stephen Pollock, MD
Vicki Saito
Robert Taber, PhD

References

Anderson, R. W. 1996. Duke University Medical Center & Health System: Accomplishments and future challenges. Duke Managed Care Education Program, Durham, N.C., 16 November.

Arnold, A. 1995. Faculty, staff discuss managed care concerns. *The Chronicle* 91:1–8 (6 December).

Bhatt, S. 1995. Medical school implements major curricular changes. *The Chronicle* 91:1–6 (6 December).

Brink, S. 1996. America's best hospitals. *US News & World Report* 121 (6): 52–87 (12 August).

Harreld, H. 1996. Study finds hospital costs high here in '94. *Triangle Business Journal* 11 (23): 4 (9 February).

N.Y. Life, Duke University form managed care joint venture. 1995. *Integrated Healthcare Report* 13 (October).

Rogers, M. C., R. Snyderman, and E. L. Rogers. 1994. Cultural and organizational implications of academic managed care networks. *New England Journal of Medicine* 331 (20): 1374–1377 (17 November).

Shortell, S. M., R. R. Gillies, D. A. Anderson, K. M. Erickson, and J. B. Mitchell. 1996. *Remaking healthcare in America: Building organized delivery systems.* San Francisco: Jossey-Bass.

Snyderman, R. 1995. Model for a 21st century academic health system. In *The Academic Health Center in 21st Century,* edited by R. Snyderman, MD, and V. Y. Saito. Durham, N.C.: Duke University Medical Center.

———. 1996. Presentation at Private Sector Conference, 15 April, at Duke University Medical Center, Durham, N.C.

Zimmer, J. 1996. Duke health plan wins mixed review. *Durham Herald,* 30 June, B1, B4.

Legal Issues Facing Integrated Delivery Systems

Eve T. Horwitz*

ecause health care executives work in one of the nation's most heavily regulated industries, they must consider the dense statutory and regulatory forest before creating or joining an integrated delivery system (IDS). This appendix explores some of the seminal legal issues managers face in the creation or modification of IDSs. It is not intended to supplant legal advice; rather, it should alert health care executives to the typical legal issues they need to consider in the development of an IDS.

This appendix focuses on some of the recurring legal questions health care executives face regarding antitrust, taxation, licensure, and other issues. Because of the differences in the type and

*Eve T. Horwitz has an independent health care legal practice in Lexington, Mass., and is of counsel to Mintz, Levin, Cohn, Ferris, Glovsky and Popeo, P.C., in Boston; she practices in the firm's health care department. She received both her JD and MBA in health care management from Boston University. Horwitz gratefully acknowledges the assistance of her colleagues Bill Coffey, Judith Lidsky, and Andy Nathanson in the preparation of this appendix.

extent of integration which occur in any single transaction or IDS model, some but not all of these issues will be germane. Additionally, some states are regulating IDSs as risk-bearing entities; health care executives should be familiar with the regulatory environment in their states.

ANTITRUST

Whenever significant actors in an industry coordinate or integrate their operations, antitrust concerns arise. By definition, an IDS results in the affiliation in some form or to some degree of two or more previously independent persons or entities. Antitrust analysis examines the effect of the integration of businesses on competition. Within an industry, integration can be horizontal, vertical, or often both. In all cases, health care managers creating an integrated system must consider the potential implication of federal as well as state antitrust laws.

Horizontal integration occurs when two or more entities providing the same service or product combine operations. The merger of two independent hospitals or the combination of two independent physician groups into an independent practice association (IPA) are examples of horizontal mergers. Vertical integration consists of the merger of two or more entities that operate at separate but complementary levels in the production or distribution chain. A physician hospital organization (PHO) is an example of vertical integration.

Because procompetitive economic efficiencies more often accompany vertical integration, regulatory agencies historically have challenged such mergers less frequently than horizontal mergers. Vertical integration can align the economic interests of previously arm's-length parties and encourage greater overall operating efficiency in delivering goods or services. For example, it may enable a manufacturer to ensure a steady source of supply in an "upstream" integration or a reliable outlet for distribution in a "downstream" merger. Similarly, vertical integration can guarantee health care providers up the service chain (like hospitals) a steady stream of business, thus affording hospitals the luxury of planning and investing for future growth confident in the knowledge that a ready market for their services will exist.[1]

Basic Antitrust Statutes

Health care managers should be aware of the antitrust principles embodied in five specific federal laws when organizing an integrated system.

Sherman Act: Section 1 Broadly drawn, section 1 of the Sherman Act prohibits "every contract, combination . . . or conspiracy" employed "in restraint" of trade. Section 1 is generally applied to concerted anticompetitive action among competitors, such as agreements to fix prices or divide markets. It is also used to challenge mergers or acquisitions.

The essence of a section 1 violation is the contract, combination, or conspiracy. With some exceptions such as tying, purely unilateral activity will not violate section 1. Thus, it is usually true that an entity such as a hospital cannot violate section 1 through "concerted" action with its own officers or employees, though many courts have created an exception for corporate officers acting on their own behalf. However, the federal courts have yet to settle the thorny question of whether a hospital can "conspire" or "combine" with its own medical staff as a whole, or with individual members of its staff. Outside the hospital arena, physicians who create an integrated group practice may be deemed incapable of conspiring or combining, but only if the practice is so truly integrated as to function as a single entity and thus constitute only one "firm."

Sherman Act: Section 2 Section 2 of the Sherman Act prohibits monopolies and conspiracies, as well as attempts to create them. This section is concerned with the development, through anticompetitive practices, of market power that enables the monopolist to artificially restrict output and inflate prices. A party acting unilaterally can violate section 2.

Based on the organization's existing market power, both product and geographic, health care executives need to consider the possible monopolistic tendencies of their integration activities. Section 2's proscription is not limited to hospital mergers that monopolize or threaten to monopolize *all* acute care services in a geographic market; it may also apply to the acquisition of market power in *sectors of services,* such as cardiac rehabilitation or pediatrics, which themselves constitute discrete "product markets."

Clayton Act: Section 7 Section 7 of the Clayton Act is the primary antitrust tool for challenging mergers and acquisitions. The statute prohibits mergers or acquisitions whose effect may be to lessen competition substantially, or to create a monopoly, for a particular product or service in a particular geographic market. Unlike sections 1 and 2 of the Sherman Act, section 7 creates a broad "incipiency" standard that can prohibit transactions that have no immediate or even imminent effect on competition. Health care executives considering joint ventures, stock or asset acquisitions, or mergers should consider the enterprise's monopolistic tendencies when structuring integration agreements. Sufficiently large transactions must be submitted to the federal government for section 7 scrutiny under the Hart-Scott-Rodino Act, discussed below.

Hart-Scott-Rodino Act The Hart-Scott-Rodino Act requires parties to certain large mergers or acquisitions to provide pre-closing notice to both the Department of Justice and the Federal Trade Commission, and to observe a mandatory waiting period while one of those agencies scrutinizes the transaction. The act is triggered when both the size of the parties involved and the size of the transaction meet statutory thresholds.[2]

During the waiting period, the reviewing agency may make a "second request" for additional information and may undertake enforcement action to block or modify the proposed transaction. Expiration of the waiting period without enforcement action does not automatically equate to antitrust "clearance," although in practice the antitrust agencies are unlikely to challenge a reported transaction unless the challenge is based on a problem that the agency had identified to the parties, or unless it concerns changed circumstances or matters that the parties failed to report to the government. Private enforcement actions by injured parties, of course, is always a possibility. Though a Hart-Scott-Rodino filing carries a steep fee of $45,000, the penalty for failing to file notification of a reportable transaction is even steeper: a fine of up to $10,000 per day.

Federal Trade Commission Act The Federal Trade Commission Act is enforced by the Federal Trade Commission (FTC). Section 5 of this statute prohibits both "unfair methods of competition" and "unfair or deceptive acts or practices." The latter clause authorizes the FTC to act as a consumer protection advocate, whereas the proscription against "unfair methods of competition" essentially gives the FTC concurrent antitrust jurisdiction with the Department of Justice. In fact, the broad language of section 5 enables the FTC to punish conduct that offends the spirit of the Sherman and Clayton Acts without technically violating their terms. Unlike the Justice Department, however, the FTC has only civil enforcement powers; it may not pursue criminal prosecutions.

Methods of Analysis

The federal courts have developed an intensely fact-specific method of antitrust analysis that requires, in each case, a careful examination of all relevant factors to determine the intent of the actors and the impact of their actions on competition. The courts have also recognized, however, that certain types of activities are so likely to be anticompetitive as to make full-blown factual scrutiny unnecessary. Consequently, there are now two methods of analysis employed by both courts and government agencies for evaluating whether business relationships violate the antitrust laws. The type of activity itself will determine which analytical framework will be applied to a particular business arrangement.

Per Se Violations   Certain business practices are deemed to be so nakedly or inherently anticompetitive that they are "per se" antitrust violations, which can be prohibited and punished without analysis of their effect on competition in particular situations. Such highly suspect activities include price fixing, group boycotts, and market division.

Price fixing: Insufficiently integrated parties will almost certainly violate antitrust law if they agree to set a certain minimum or maximum market price for goods or a service. Separate entities within a partially integrated system that agree to certain fee schedules may also be at risk under the antitrust laws; that risk may be reduced if they are in global or other capitated arrangements.

Group boycotts: Group boycotts of a particular market participant can also result in an antitrust violation when the purpose of the exclusion is anticompetitive in nature. As an example, an IPA that refuses to affiliate with a particular group practice in an attempt to prevent that group from competing in the market may run afoul of antitrust law. On the other hand, affiliation standards may become so inclusive as to create monopolistic tendencies that may expose the group to attack for violations of section 2 of the Sherman Act. Unfortunately, in most circumstances there are few "bright lines" assisting health care executives in evaluating when an integrated system wields monopoly power. Circumstances need to be evaluated on a case-by-case basis.

Market division: Competitors violate antitrust law when they purposely divide the market among themselves. As with other per se violations of the antitrust laws, the intent of the parties—or even whether market division has a procompetitive purpose—is irrelevant.

Covenants not to compete: Far less likely to fall into the realm of per se violations are covenants not to compete. In general, covenants not to compete are treated under state common law as legitimate business practices, properly employed to protect the business interests of parties to an agreement as long as the restrictions they impose are reasonably limited. In creating covenants not to compete, therefore, managers should ensure that the geographic and durational scope of the covenants meet applicable standards of reasonableness. They should also note that some states view covenants not to compete in physician contracts as violations of public policy, and thus unenforceable.

Rule of Reason   If an activity does not constitute a per se violation of the antitrust laws, it may still be illegal under the *rule of reason* analysis. Under the rule of reason, courts examine a number of factors to determine whether an activity is unreasonably anticompetitive, including the purpose of the integration, each party's market share, and the estimated competitive effects of the integration. The rule of reason analysis requires a complex and often speculative review of a delivery system's procompetitive and anticompetitive tendencies. The examiner depends on a number of factual assumptions and, as a result, rule of reason cases can become very detailed. For example, an assessment of a party's market share will depend on the definition of the product and the market. Such a determination may require calculation of all eligible patients in a certain geographic area, broken down by patients covered by certain insurance provisions or those requiring particular services within the "market" area. Obviously, the definition and determination of both product (for example, HMO coverage versus all health insurance) and geographic market will be very important to the analysis.

Antitrust Implications of Integration Activities

The advent of managed care has resulted in widespread restructuring throughout the health care industry. Increased competition for finite health care dollars has seen the industry undertake numerous health care mergers, acquisitions, and affiliations.

For antitrust purposes, the primary issue involving these newly created entities is whether their merger represents full or merely partial integration. If sufficient integration exists, courts will permit the transaction under a rule of reason standard as long as the relationship does not constitute an unduly burdensome restraint of trade or consolidation of market power.

In the case of a merger or acquisition, once full integration occurs, the entity becomes a single entity, unable to conspire with itself to restrain trade. The issue of full versus partial integration is more complicated in an affiliation arrangement.

Partially integrated enterprises such as PHOs or IPAs raise questions as to whether such entities are entitled to engage in concerted action that would otherwise contravene various federal and state antitrust statutes. As stated previously, antitrust analysis is usually very fact-specific. Thus, any definition of a sufficiently integrated health care system would be, at best, amorphous. Antitrust regulators, however, are more likely to look favorably on those business enterprises in which partners do the following:

- Share joint control
- Share economic and capital risk
- Offer a new product to the market or facilitate the entry of new competitors to the market
- Separate the enterprise from the partners

Additionally, the partners should permit the fledgling enterprise to do the following:

- Control the means of production and procurement of supplies
- Centralize operations at a common location
- Earn and collect its own revenues and conduct its own administrative functions

- Perform its own credentialing, utilization review, and quality assurance programs
- Market itself as an individual entity
- Employ its own staff and offer its own employee benefits package

When a significant number of these factors are present in a new enterprise, regulators are more likely to conclude that economic integration exists and to apply the less onerous rule of reason analysis.

Federal Enforcement Policy

Recognizing the emerging prominence of antitrust issues in the business of health care, the Department of Justice and the FTC in 1993 and 1994 issued significant enforcement policy statements concerning antitrust law and the health care industry. The agencies updated these statements in 1996. In the policy statements, the agencies created "safety zones" that permit certain cooperative activities among health care entities without invoking antitrust investigation. These "safety zones" include the following:

- Hospital mergers between two general acute care hospitals when one hospital is at least five years old, has fewer than 100 licensed beds, and a daily average inpatient census of less than 40.
- Hospital joint ventures involving high-technology or other expensive equipment, if the venture includes only the number of hospitals whose participation is needed to support the equipment. The safety zone covers both new and existing equipment. Typical joint ventures protected by this safety zone would include cooperative purchases of magnetic resonance imaging or computerized tomography equipment.
- Providers' collective provision of outcome data to purchasers. This is recognized and protected as a legitimate means of improving the quality and efficiency of patient care, as long as the information is used for that, and not some anticompetitive, purpose.
- Providers' collective disclosure of price and cost information to purchasers. This is also protected within a safety

zone as long as the information is sufficiently diluted and collected by third parties. Current price information may not be shared among providers, nor may any other information unless there are at least five providers reporting data, and no single provider's contribution represents more than 25 percent of the data sample.

- Joint purchasing arrangements among health care providers, as long as the purchases account for less than 35 percent of sales in the relevant market, and the cost for each participant is less than 20 percent of its total annual revenues.

- Nonexclusive physician network joint ventures, as long as the physician participants share substantial financial risk (for example, through a capitation arrangement), and no more than 30 percent of the physicians within each specialty in the geographic market join the venture.

- Exclusive network joint ventures, as long as the physician participants share substantial financial risk, and no more than 20 percent of the specialty physicians with active hospital privileges in the geographic market join the venture.

Sanctions

Health care executives can face antitrust challenges from any number of fronts, including the Department of Justice and the FTC on the federal level, state attorneys general, and private litigants. Private litigants under the Sherman or Clayton Acts or state antitrust laws may be awarded treble damages and attorney fees. Although most antitrust actions are civil, the federal government can and does criminally prosecute Sherman Act violations, particularly those it considers "blatant" violations of per se proscriptions. The maximum statutory penalty under sections 1 and 2 of the Sherman Act is a corporate fine of $10 million and an individual fine of $350,000 and/or up to three years in prison. However, criminal fines can exceed even those amounts where there are multiple violations (each subject to the statutory maximum), or where the offender is punished under federal sentencing guidelines, under the authority of an alternative sentencing statute that imposes a fine of up to twice the pecuniary gain or loss caused by the antitrust violation.

In addition, courts may impose other penalties, including mandatory divestiture, injunctions, and consent decrees prohibiting

certain activity. It is obviously imperative that a health care executive embarking on integration activities be aware of the antitrust
considerations in such endeavors.

FRAUD AND ABUSE LAWS

As with the antitrust laws, health care executives evaluating
involvement in an integrated system need to be sensitive to the
fraud and abuse laws. In an IDS context, these laws may be most
relevant to physician relationships.

Numerous federal and state laws concerning health care
providers' referral of patients fall under the umbrella of "fraud and
abuse." Pertinent statutes include the federal anti-kickback law concerning government health programs (the anti-kickback statute), the
federal ban on physician referrals to institutions in which the physician or an immediate family member holds an investment interest or
has a compensation arrangement (the Stark law), and the federal
Medicare and Medicaid False Claims Act. Because Medicare and Medicaid make up such a large percentage of the nation's health care budget, and because the civil and criminal penalties are so severe,
considerations of the federal self-referral laws, especially the anti-kickback statute, should permeate every health care executive's decision-
making process. Additionally, most states have anti-kickback,
anti-self-referral, fee-splitting, or other similar laws that may extend
the federal prohibitions to all payers or health care providers.

Federal Anti-Kickback Law

With the passage of the 1996 Health Insurance Portability and
Accountability Act (HIPAA), anti-kickback provisions that previously applied only to Medicare and Medicaid funds have been
greatly expanded to cover any federal health benefits program
except for the Federal Employees Health Benefit Program.

In very broad language, the anti-kickback statute prohibits
providers of covered services or goods from knowingly and will-
fully soliciting, receiving or providing any remuneration, directly or
indirectly, in cash or in kind, in exchange for either referring an
individual, or furnishing or arranging a good or service for which
payment may be made by any federal health care program.

Although the language of the anti-kickback statute is expansive, it does contain numerous statutory exceptions, including discounts for employees. In 1987, Congress mandated that the Office of Inspector General (OIG) of the Department of Health and Human Services adopt regulatory "safe harbors," which have the effect of exempting parties from criminal prosecution or exclusion from any federal health care program under the law's provisions. The safe harbors, however, do not shield parties from prosecution under any other federal or state law prohibiting referrals or bribery.

The areas in which some of the most significant safe harbor protection has been provided include investment interests, rental agreements, personal service and management contracts, employees, practice acquisition, referral services, group purchasing and volume discounts, and risk-sharing arrangements.

Investment Interests   Executives must use caution when structuring investment interests in health care facilities. Although ownership of a management services organization (MSO) limited only to administrative or business guidance generally will not violate the anti-kickback statute if no patient contact occurs, any ownership structure that influences the volume of business may well violate the statute. The safe harbor for small entities applies if no more than 40 percent of the investment interests are held by investors who provide services or create business for the entity, while a safe harbor for rural providers expands the allowance to 75 percent.

Rental Agreements   The rental safe harbor allows integrated systems to lease office space and equipment to providers without contravening the anti-kickback statute. To fall within the safe harbor, the rental agreement must, among other requirements, be for fair market value and be for a minimum of one year. Executives must be vigilant in ensuring that all transactions with providers represent fair market value, as the fair market value requirement is a cornerstone of the anti-kickback statute. Equally important, fair market valuations may not take into consideration the potential value of referrals or the site's proximity to a referral source. Executives considering rental agreements with providers should always secure an independent fair market appraisal before entering into lease agreements.

Personal Service and Management Contracts   To come under the safe harbors, personal service and management agreements must be at least one year in length and represent fair market value payment not based on the value or volume of referred services. Part-time contracts must include the schedule of service intervals and the exact length and charge for each service interval. As in the rental agreements, fair market valuations may not take into consideration proximity to potential referral sources.

Employees The employee safe harbor covers employer payments to providers in a bona fide employment relationship. Although the employee exception provides employers with some leeway in establishing compensation packages for its provider employees, employers should be wary when considering the award of bonuses based on referral volume. Additionally, prudent management practice suggests executives should put in writing employment agreements with employees to eliminate ambiguity in any safe harbor determination.

Practice Acquisition Although the practice acquisition safe harbor applies only to sales between practitioners, unofficial declarations from the OIG acknowledge that acquisition of physician practices by an integrated system are permissible as long as the parties base the transactions on the practice's fair market value and exclude any referral value. As a practical matter, health care executives should always obtain independent appraisals confirming the fair market value of a transaction before entering into agreements.

Referral Services Integrated systems must follow fairly detailed requirements to fall within the safe harbor for physician referral services. Under the safe harbor, referral services may not exclude any provider that meets the system's participation requirements, nor may the system discriminate in its application of referral criteria among participating providers. Additionally, the safe harbor requires full disclosure to persons seeking referrals from the service of how the referral service selects its providers, collectively and individually, whether the referral service receives a fee (which may not exceed the cost of operating the service), the relationship between the provider and the service, and restrictions that would exclude a provider.

Group Purchasing and Volume Discounts The concern with group purchasing discounts is that volume discounts may easily masquerade as referral bonuses. As a result, the statute and regulations require parties to link the time of the transaction. In addition, the discount must be disclosed and reflected in the provider's claims submission.

Risk-Sharing Arrangements   HIPAA created a new safe harbor that applies to written agreements involving remuneration between organizations and individuals or entities in two circumstances. In the first instance, the organization must be a federally certified HMO or competitive medical plan. In the second, the risk-sharing arrangement must place the individual or entity at substantial financial risk for the cost or utilization of items or services the provider is obligated to produce.[3]

In addition to the enacted safe harbors, the OIG published a number of proposed safe harbors. Although these were never formally adopted, they provide substantial guidance on the OIG's likely interpretations of the fraud and abuse statutes. They include the following:

- Investment interests in group practices
- Investment interests in rural areas
- Investment interests in ambulatory surgical centers
- Referral arrangements for specialty services
- Rural physician recruitment
- Obstetrical malpractice insurance subsidies
- Cooperative hospital services organizations
- Volume discounts
- Sham transactions

OIG Enforcement

Although full compliance with a safe harbor immunizes parties from criminal or civil prosecution, it is not necessarily true that an arrangement that falls outside the safe harbors is criminally or civilly suspect. Executives entering agreements among health care providers should always attempt to mirror the requirements of applicable safe harbor provisions, keeping in mind that the OIG could still find as valid agreements that stray outside regulatory requirements.

One of the more significant provisions of HIPAA requires the OIG, for the first four years after the enactment of the statute, to issue advisory opinions regarding fraud and abuse concerns. For example, parties to a transaction could solicit the OIG's opinion as to whether a particular proposed arrangement would satisfy the requirements of an exception to the anti-kickback statute. This requirement may be helpful to a hospital considering an integration arrangement but desiring the comfort of prior approval by the OIG with respect to fraud and abuse concerns. HIPAA specifically exempts fair market value and bona fide employment issues from the mandatory advisory opinion requirements. Under the statute, the OIG must issue its advisory opinion within 60 days of receipt, although executives should note that the Clinton administration, in conjunction with its reservations on the new risk-sharing arrangement safe harbor, has expressed its desire that Congress repeal the mandatory advisory opinion provision. Further, HIPAA requires the OIG to create new safe harbors that consider access, quality, patient freedom of choice, competition, potential overutilization, and cost of federal health care programs.

In addition to the recently mandated advisory opinions, the OIG voluntarily issues periodic fraud alerts concerning burgeoning or recurrent activities it believes contravene the law. These fraud alerts contain numerous issues for the IDS executive.

The OIG issued its first fraud alert in 1989, outlining joint venture characteristics it considered suspect. These included arrangements with the following elements:

- Incentive programs reward provider investors for referring patients.
- Provider investors are likely to serve as a significant referral source.
- Referral information is tracked and distributed to investors.
- Provider investors are encouraged to refer to the entity or divest their holdings in the entity if referrals fail to meet "acceptable" levels.
- Provider investors' change in status is linked to referral capabilities.
- Provider investors' investment return far outweighs investment risk.
- Provider investors are allowed to borrow their capital contributions from their joint venture partner and then repay it through deductions from profit distributions.

In 1991, the OIG issued a fraud alert concerning the waiver of patient co-payment and deductibles under Medicare part B. The

OIG theorized that the payments are inducements to attract business and encourage patients to make health care choices based on financial, rather than medical, considerations. Later in 1991, the OIG warned against municipalities soliciting contracts with private ambulance companies.

In 1992, the OIG issued a significant fraud alert concerning hospital incentives to physicians. Suspect incentive payments include:

- The use of free or significantly discounted office space or equipment, particularly facilities located close to the hospital
- Payment of any sort of incentive by the hospital for patient referrals
- Provision of free or significantly discounted billing, nursing, or staff services
- Free training for a physician's office staff in such areas as management techniques, CPT coding, and laboratory techniques
- Guarantees that if a physician's income fails to reach a predetermined level, the hospital will supplement the remainder up to a certain amount
- Low-interest or interest-free loans, or loans that may be forgiven if a physician refers patients (or some number of patients) to the hospital
- Payment of a physician's travel costs and expenses associated with conferences
- Payment for a physician's continuing education courses
- Coverage under the hospital's group health insurance plans at an inappropriate low cost to the physician
- Payment for services, including consultations at the hospital, that require few, if any, substantive duties by the physician, or payment in excess of fair market value of services rendered

A 1994 fraud alert from the OIG warned the public about potential fraudulent implications when drug companies offer payments to physicians in exchange for physicians' agreeing to prescribe certain pharmaceutical products.

In 1995, the OIG issued two more fraud alerts. The first fraud alert concerned the rapidly growing segments of the health care industry devoted to home health care. The OIG is particularly concerned with the following suspicious practices:

- Claims for home health visits that were never made and for visits to ineligible beneficiaries
- Fraud in annual cost report claims
- Paying or receiving kickbacks in exchange for Medicare or Medicaid referrals
- Marketing uncovered or unneeded home care services to beneficiaries

The second 1995 fraud alert concerned fraud and abuse in the provision of medical supplies to nursing facilities. The OIG is wary of the following practices:

- Claims for medical supplies and equipment that are not medically necessary
- Claims for items that are not provided as claimed or are double-billed
- Payment or receiving kickbacks in exchange for Medicare or Medicaid referrals
- Claims for delivery of unordered goods
- Nursing home solicitation of unauthorized deliveries in exchange for access to patient's medical records and other information needed to bill Medicare

Sanctions

Violation of the anti-kickback statute subjects transgressors to numerous civil and criminal penalties, many of which were broadened and heightened under HIPAA.

In addition to criminal convictions that can result in prison sentences of up to five years and fines of $25,000, the anti-kickback statute contains mandatory exclusions from continuing participation for parties convicted of felonies pertaining to federal health care programs and permissive exclusions for parties convicted of certain misdemeanors. Also, HIPAA increases the maximum civil money penalty amounts from $2,000 to $10,000 per violation while increasing the maximum assessment by 50 percent from double the amount claimed to triple the amount claimed. Furthermore, health care executives should note that HIPAA authorizes the exclusion of individuals with a direct or indirect controlling interest in a sanctioned entity where the individual knew or should have known of the illicit activity or where the individual was an officer or managing employee of the entity.

Finally, executives should be aware that along with the recently increased penalties comes a correlative increase in enforcement capabilities; the Federal Bureau of Investigation (FBI) has placed a renewed emphasis on prosecuting health care crimes, evidenced by the exponential growth in prosecuted cases in the 1990s. Congress has responded to the FBI's vigor in investigating fraud and abuse by providing the agency with additional funding that has permitted the FBI to significantly increase its presence in the field.

Self-Referral Prohibitions

Initially adopted as the Ethics and Patient Referrals Act of 1989, and expanded by statute as part of the Omnibus Reconciliation Act of 1993, the federal statute prohibiting physician self-referral is commonly known as Stark, named for its primary author, Rep. Fourtney "Pete" Stark. The original statute, "Stark I," prohibited physician referrals to clinical laboratories if they had an ownership interest in the laboratory; "Stark II," the 1993 amendment, expanded the prohibitions to a broad array of health care services. Stark has significant implications for vertically integrated IDSs because it broadly restricts Medicare and Medicaid reimbursement for services provided as a result of physician referrals to entities with which the physician has a "financial relationship."

Stark prohibits physician referral for certain designated health services (DHS) if the physician (or immediate family member) has a financial interest in the entity to which the patient is referred. Similarly, an institution will not be paid for claims if they were for services generated by prohibited referrals. Like the anti-kickback statute, however, Stark contains exceptions for specific financial relationships and services. Unlike the anti-kickback statute, Stark requires no criminal intent to contravene the statute to create a violation. The mere existence of a DHS referral to an entity in which an improper financial relationship exists creates an automatic Stark violation.

When considering potential Stark implications of their business arrangements, health care executives must understand the following:

- What constitutes a DHS under the statute
- The "financial relationships" between the IDS, its physicians, and providers of DHSs as they apply to Stark

- The limited exceptions to general prohibitions on self-referral
- The potential penalties associated with Stark violations

Designated Health Services Under Stark, a financially interested physician, or the entity with which the physician has a financial interest, may not submit a Medicare or Medicaid bill for any of the following services:

- Clinical laboratory services
- Radiology services, including magnetic resonance imaging, computer axial tomography, and ultrasound services
- Radiation therapy services and supplies
- Physical and occupational therapy services
- Durable medical equipment and supplies
- Parenteral and enteral nutrients, equipment, and supplies
- Prosthetics, orthotics, and prosthetic devices and supplies
- Outpatient prescription drugs
- Home health services
- Inpatient and outpatient hospital services

Not included as DHSs in the 1993 expansion of Stark (thus not subject to Stark penalties) are such services as the following:

- Ambulatory surgical facility services if provided by a hospital
- Home infusion therapy services
- Home dialysis services
- Ambulance services
- Vision correction products
- Comprehensive outpatient rehabilitation facilities services

Financial Relationship Stark defines "financial relationship" as a direct or indirect relationship between a physician (or a member of a physician's immediate family) and an entity in which the physician or family member has an ownership or investment interest or a compensation arrangement. Consequently, under Stark, either investment relationships or compensation arrangements will trigger the act's applicability. Health care executives must be aware, however, of the Stark exceptions that are distinct from those that exist under the anti-kickback statute. Furthermore, executives must be able to distinguish between Stark's compensation and investment exceptions.

Investment Interest Exceptions   In addition to investments in well-capitalized (greater than $75 million) public corporations or mutual funds or other regulated investment companies, Stark includes limited exceptions for ownership or investment interests in the following entities:

- Hospitals in Puerto Rico
- Certain rural providers
- Hospital-provided DHSs when the referring physician has authorized privileges at the hospital and an ownership interest in the entire hospital and not just one of its subdivisions
- Hospitals outside Puerto Rico where a medical staff member's ownership interest does not relate to a DHS

Compensation Arrangement Exceptions   Unless certain requirements are met, Stark prohibits compensation arrangements—defined as including the payment of any remuneration, directly or indirectly, overtly or covertly, in cash or in kind—between physicians or members of their immediate families, and entities except for the following:

- Any compensation arrangement with a hospital that does not relate to the provision of designated health services
- An arrangement between an employer and a physician (or immediate family member) for the bona fide employment of the physician (or family member)
- Remuneration from an entity under a personal service arrangement, including a physician incentive plan
- Remuneration provided by a hospital to induce a physician to relocate to the hospital's geographic area
- Payments made for the rental or lease of office space and equipment
- An isolated financial transaction, such as the one-time sale of property
- Payment by a physician to a laboratory in exchange for services, or to an entity as compensation for other items or services at a price consistent with fair market value
- An arrangement in existence since 1989 between a hospital and a group under which designated health services are provided by the group but are billed by the hospital

Exceptions Applicable to Compensation Arrangements and Investment Interests   A final hybrid category of exceptions applies to both compensation arrangements and investment interests, including the following:

- Physician services provided personally by another physician in the same group practice of the referring physician
- Services furnished by a prepaid plan or other HMO as defined by the statute
- In-office ancillary services provided by the referring physician or persons in the physician's group practice, if certain detailed requirements are met

The group practice exception regulations require that group member physicians furnish and bill 75 percent of total patient services through the group.

Sanctions

Entities providing DHS services must report to the Health Care Financing Administration (HCFA) all physicians who have an ownership or investment interest in the entity. Failure to comply with the registration requirement can subject the entity to a civil money penalty of up to $10,000 a day. Stark violations carry a mandatory penalty denying reimbursement for services rendered or a refund of any amounts billed and collected for the inappropriate treatment. The OIG may also impose civil monetary penalties of up to $15,000 for each prohibited referral for which a bill was submitted and up to $100,000 for an entity that enters into a "circumvention scheme." More significantly, parties that violate Stark are subject to treble damages and exclusion from participation in the Medicare and Medicaid programs. Because IDSs often create complex, multitiered relationships, health care executives must have a working knowledge of Stark and its implications. The mere existence of only two common IDS elements gives rise to potential Stark problems: a physician referral and a designated health service.

At the outset, health care executives should realize that the Stark exception for isolated transactions may immunize physician practice acquisitions from Stark prosecution. Nonetheless, executives should be careful about the manner in which they consummate such transactions. In 1995, the OIG stated that physician practice acquisitions financed by installment payments would not find safe harbor in the isolated transaction exception. Because the employee exception allows only for payments to physicians at the fair market value of physician services, health care executives must tread carefully when making financial arrangements for physician practice acquisitions. Once an IDS is up and running, Stark provides several exceptions that protect physician payments, ranging from the employee exception to personal service arrangements. Nevertheless, these compensation arrangements must be structured carefully in order not to contravene Stark self-referral prohibitions.

False Claims Act

In addition to the federal laws prohibiting illegal remuneration and self-referral, the successful manager must be aware of the legal pitfalls associated with false or fraudulent billing. Under the federal False Claims Act, any person who knowingly presents, or causes to be presented, a false or fraudulent claim for payment or approval, or conspires to defraud the government by getting a false or fraudulent claim allowed or paid, faces severe punitive liability.

The statute subjects those who violate the False Claims Act to civil damages of between $5,000 and $10,000 for each false or fraudulent claim; the statute then trebles the damages. Civil cases under the statute often involve hundreds or thousands of false claims, exposing health care entities to potentially enormous damages. Onerous False Claims Act penalties have the practical result of forcing defendants to settle rather than face potentially bankrupting judgments. Since 1995, settlements of False Claims Act claims have run into the tens of millions of dollars.

Complicating matters for health care executives is the "bounty" element within the False Claims Act that rewards private citizens who initiate on behalf of the government qui tam litigation against parties submitting false claims. Qui tam plaintiffs are entitled to 15 percent of any damage award judgment if the government decides to intervene, and 25 percent if the government does not. Qui tam actions are often brought by competitors' employees or past or even current employees within the organization against whom false claims are charged.

Recent settlements worked out by the Department of Justice suggests several billing practices to which health care executives should pay careful attention. These include cases involving suspect billing for the following:

- Investigational or experimental devices for which the government has yet to give its approval
- Diagnosis-related group services provided within 72 hours of a patient's inpatient admission to a hospital as non-physician outpatient treatment
- Faculty physician services at teaching hospitals
- "Unbundled" laboratory tests

The dual threats of government and private action require health care executives to develop comprehensive "corporate compliance programs." In doing so, proactive managers can minimize inaccurate billing practices before they become systemic. Additionally, under federal sentencing guidelines, courts may reduce minimum penalties for those entities found to have corporate compliance programs in place. It is imperative that managers of health care entities vigilantly monitor their claims practice and respond quickly to potentially fraudulent activity. The potential exposure for an executive embarking on IDS initiatives (for example, in the acquisition of a physician practice with inaccurate billing practices) can be substantial.

TAXATION

Qualifying for Tax Exemption

IDS formation gives rise to a number of federal and state tax issues. Historically, hospitals have chosen to operate as tax-exempt non-profit organizations, while the vast majority of individual physicians and physician group practices have operated as for-profit enterprises. The integration of entities with such disparate missions creates a number of important tax issues for the health care manager.

Section 501(c)(3) of the Internal Revenue Code (IRC) grants tax-exempt status to those corporations organized and operated exclusively for religious, charitable, scientific, literary, or educational purposes. The Internal Revenue Service (IRS) has long recognized the nonprofit promotion of health as a charitable purpose.

Over time, the IRS has expanded the concept of health promotion to encompass nonprofit organizations other than hospitals that promote the health of the community. However, the IRS generally does not grant exemption to IPAs and MSOs. The IRS's view is that these entities operate primarily to benefit private physicians. A clinic, however, if operated on a nonprofit basis and with proper safeguards, can qualify for exemption.

A for-profit component of an IDS can qualify for tax exemption if it is nonprofit and provides medical care by employing or contracting with physicians or if it operates in support of an organization that provides such care. The basis for exemption lies in the traditional standards applied to hospitals. To qualify for exemption, hospitals must meet a "community benefit" standard. Hospitals satisfy the community benefit requirement of the IRS if they maintain the following:

- An emergency room open to everyone regardless of ability to pay
- Non-emergency-room services without regard to the patient's chosen method of payment, including Medicare or Medicaid
- An open medical staff
- A policy against patient dumping
- A board of directors that represents a broad cross-section of the community

Hospitals within an IDS must satisfy all the above. Nonhospitals seeking tax exemption must satisfy all relevant requirements and are generally asked to demonstrate a strong commitment to charity care and other community benefits such as improved delivery of care and increased accessibility of care. In this era of integration, IDS executives must ensure that they do not jeopardize their enterprise's tax-exempt status by creating improper corporate structures.

Community board membership requirements can be extremely vexing. Unfortunately for health care executives, issues of board membership are among the most significant factors the IRS considers when granting tax-exempt status. The IRS mandates that disinterested members of the community control hospital boards on the grounds that financially interested parties may pursue private interests ahead of the facility's tax-exempt mission. Nevertheless, in 1993 the IRS granted a 20 percent safe harbor for board participation by financially interested physicians. Just three years later, in July 1996, the IRS liberalized the safe harbor; now up to 49 percent of a tax-exempt entity's board may comprise interested parties, provided that certain conflict-of-interest criteria are met. Although the IRS has not specifically delineated to whom the new safe harbor applies, it is certain that physicians compensated by the tax-exempt facility— as well as officers, department heads, and employees of the facility—are subject to the restriction. This new 49 percent safe harbor also applies to committees with board-delegated powers.

Executives should note that the new liberalized board allowances have fairly detailed two instances where IRS policy permits deviation from the 49 percent rule. The IRS will allow unlimited physician participation in clinical or professional committees. In contrast, committees on physician compensation must not have participation by interested physicians. The IRS insists on complete independence of physician compensation committees to prevent inappropriate physician enrichment in contravention of the organization's tax-exempt purpose.

Specifically, the IRS model conflict of interest policy requires exempt organizations to do the following:

- Identify interested persons including directors, officers, persons in positions of influence, and persons with direct or indirect financial interests
- Require interested persons to disclose potential and actual conflicts under penalty of discipline or corrective action
- Determine if a true conflict exists by means of a vote of disinterested directors
- Investigate alternative arrangements by means of a vote of a disinterested board of directors for the most advantageous, fair, and reasonable transaction
- Require annual statements from all directors, principal officers, and members of committees with board-delegated powers affirming their receipt, understanding, and agreement to comply with the conflict-of-interest policy
- Conduct periodic reviews of the benefits and compensation, joint ventures, partnerships and acquisitions, and contracts to determine if they are (i) reasonable, (ii) the result of arm's-length negotiations, (iii) furthering a charitable purpose, and (iv) not resulting in private inurement or impermissible private benefit

Unrelated Business Income The failure of the new IDS construct to neatly mesh with the old charitable hospital construct goes beyond issues of corporate governance. Executives engaging in IDS development must be aware of merger and acquisition activity that may endanger those tax-exempt components of the IDS. The IRS will consider an entity exclusively operated for an exempt purpose only if it "primarily" operates in furtherance of exempt purposes. In other words, a tax-exempt organization's unrelated activities may constitute no more than an "insubstantial part" of its total activity.

The IRS has not placed a numerical or percentage value on its definition of "primarily," leaving uncertainty as to how much nonexempt activity will jeopardize an entity's tax-exempt status. Unrelated businesses that result in substantial income are often spun off into separate taxable subsidiaries within the IDS. A 501(c)(3) organization may be a shareholder in a taxable corporation without having taxable activities attributed to it, unless the tax-exempt organization has not only a controlling interest but also ongoing day-to-day management of the taxable corporation's affairs.

In contrast, participation in a joint venture or a limited liability corporation (LLC) is riskier. These arrangements are generally treated as partnerships for federal tax purposes, although this may change somewhat as the IRS develops its position on LLCs. The activities of a partnership are proportionately attributed to its partners. If a tax-exempt organization is a limited partner, the IRS generally treats the activity as an investment; therefore, the investment must make economic sense and should be profitable. A 501(c)(3) organization can be a general partner only if the partnership activity is related.

Tax-exempt organizations must report to the IRS unrelated activity income on annual information returns; the returns are subject to IRS audit. In determining whether an organization has engaged in too much activity unrelated to its exempt purpose, the IRS is authorized to conduct a rather broad review, examining the organization's revenues, expenses, time and capital expenditures, resources, and office space associated with all activity, exempt and nonexempt. Income from those activities that are unrelated to the organization's exempt purpose is called unrelated business income (UBI) and is taxed at the standard corporate taxation rate.

UBI is defined as any income from trade or business regularly carried on by the organization that is not substantially related to the organization's exempt purpose. Activities conducted by volunteers or engaged in for the convenience of patients and employees are not treated as "unrelated." According to government regulations, an activity is "substantially" related to an exempt purpose for UBI purposes when the activity "contributes importantly" to the accomplishment of an exempt purpose. Although the IRS has not created a "bright line" rule defining the meaning of the term *contributes importantly*, it has definitively ruled on several hospital businesses that it considers sufficiently related to a hospital's exempt function, including the following:

- The operation of a gift shop for patients, visitors making purchases for patients, and employees
- The operation of a cafeteria/coffee shop for employees and medical staff
- The operation of a parking lot for patients and visitors
- The sale of pharmaceuticals to its patients ("patients" does not include sales to private patients of physicians who have offices in a medical building owned by a hospital)
- The performance of pathological diagnostic tests by a teaching hospital for patients of its medical staff
- The sale of durable medical equipment
- The rental of pagers to staff doctors
- The leasing of space in a medical office building if the lease enhances the use of diagnostic facilities, facilitates patient admissions, increases the availability of physicians for duty, and enhances their participation in medical education and research programs

Even if UBI is found, the IRS modifies the taxation of certain kinds of UBI. "Passive" forms of income, including the following, are not taxed:

- Dividends
- Interest in annuities, unless derived from a "controlled" corporation
- Rents from real, personal, and debt-financed property under certain circumstances

Private Inurement and Benefits A tax-exempt organization fails to satisfy the exclusivity of purpose requirements whenever the fruits of its operation inure to the benefit of private parties.

A tax-exempt organization can avoid forfeiting its tax-exempt status if it can show that any private benefit resulting from its operations is merely "incidental" to a public purpose and "insubstantial" to the private party.

Health care executives can ensure that private benefits associated with a transaction are merely incidental by demonstrating that a necessary relationship exists between the hospital's exempt purpose and the means chosen to achieve the goal. The IRS analyzes whether the activity is necessary to achieve the hospital's exempt purpose and whether the private party is merely a fortuitous beneficiary of a necessary byproduct of the transaction.

In addition to establishing the "qualitative" incidental nature of the transaction, parties attempting to justify the private enrichment derived from a tax-exempt activity must demonstrate that the benefit conferred was "quantitatively" no greater than necessary to achieve the organization's exempt purpose. The IRS generally reviews the proportionality of questionable transactions by measuring the costs of an activity against the activity's benefits to the organization and community in general.

Health care executives can deflect undesirable IRS attention and protect their tax-exempt status by documenting their decision-making processes. Executives of tax-exempt hospitals should document that the following occurred:

- Negotiations were conducted at arm's length
- Limits were placed on the hospital's potential risk or investment
- The hospital retains control over conduct of the activity or at least in proportion to its investment
- Payments and investment returns to private individuals are limited to reasonable amounts

A subset of private benefit—inurement to "insiders"—is subject to exceptional scrutiny and harsh treatment by the IRS.

The IRS has expanded its definition of *insider for private benefit purposes* to broadly include all persons with an economic relationship with, or personal or private interest in, the exempt organization. It generally considers all physicians to be "insiders." Although the private benefit test does not serve as a prohibition on all transactions, it places a stringent burden of proof on tax-exempt organizations and individuals engaging in insider transactions. Essentially, the IRS requires all such transactions to be conducted on commercially reasonable terms; this stipulation generally requires arm's-length dealings resulting in fair market valuations. In the IDS context, particular pressure points exist when hospital funds are used to capitalize MSOs or PHOs or are used to purchase physician practices.

Sanctions

Until recently, the only sanction for violation of the private inurement prohibition or public benefit requirement was revocation of tax-exempt status. In July 1996, however, the "Taxpayer Bill of Rights II" became law. This statute enables the IRS to impose intermediate sanctions such as excise taxes, rather than the extreme of revoking tax-exempt status, for violations of the private inurement prohibition.

The statute applies to transactions involving an excess benefit. Excess benefit is defined as economic benefit exceeding the consideration, including the performance of services received for providing such benefit. The statute imposes a two-tier tax upon "disqualified" persons, described as the following:

- Any person who was, at any time during the five-year period ending on the date of the excess benefit transaction, in a position to exercise substantial influence over the affairs of the organization
- A member of the family of an individual described above
- Any entity for which such person or such person's family member has a 35 percent voting power, profit interest, or beneficial interest, as determined by using constructive ownership provisions

The first-tier tax on illegal transactions is the equivalent of 25 percent of the excess benefit. The second-tier tax permits the IRS to confiscate 200 percent of the excess benefit if the excess benefit is not "corrected" before the earlier of the date the notice of deficiency was mailed or an initial tax was imposed. Health care executives should note that Congress specifically stated that physicians will be considered insiders only if they are in a position to exercise substantial influence.

The statute also imposes a single-tier tax on "organization managers"—defined as any officer, director, or trustee of the exempt organization, or any individual having similar powers—unless the organization manager's participation in a transaction is not willful and is due to reasonable cause. The tax imposed on the organization manager is 10 percent of the excess benefit. There is a $10,000 cap for each excess benefit transaction.

The statute does not impose a tax on the exempt organization itself. However, the exempt organization cannot reimburse the disqualified persons or organization managers for excess taxes imposed on them or purchase liability insurance for them unless the reimbursement or purchase falls within the limits of reasonable compensation. Executives should note that the statute applies retroactively to excess benefit transactions occurring on or after September 14, 1995. It is expected that regulations will establish a rebutable presumption of a transaction's reasonableness if it is approved by an independent board or committee, is well-documented, and meets certain other requirements. Additionally, managers should note that the statute imposes additional filing and public disclosure requirements and corresponding penalties.

Lobbying and Political Activity   The final significant area where tax-exempt entities can create trouble for themselves concerns lobbying and political activity. Exempt organizations may in no way support the election of individual political candidates. With respect to general political activity, exempt organizations must follow rules similar to the general requirement for tax-exempt status in that exempt organizations may engage in no more than an "insubstantial" amount of political activity intended to effect legislation. As in other areas of tax law, the term "insubstantial" is ambiguously defined, and it is unclear how the IRS measures an organization's political activity. A likely scenario has the IRS looking at such things as expenditures for political activity, the importance of the activity to the political cause, and the number of hours devoted to the activity by the organization. Alternatively, the organization can elect to have its lobbying activity measured by a specific percentage of its expenditures, subject to a cap.

Tax-exempt Bonds   For tax-exempt organizations with outstanding tax-exempt bonds or organizations considering new tax-exempt financing, particular guidelines must be adhered to in the IDS context. For example, there is a $150 million cap on the amount of outstanding tax-exempt bonds a group of affiliates may issue for nonhospital facilities such as nursing homes.

As another example, use of bond-financed facilities for unrelated business or by private persons is very limited. Often, problems with management or service contracts (which would include contracts for physician and other professional services) can be avoided if the contracts contain certain compensation restrictions and limitations on term. However, there are also limitations on related party contracts. These could be stumbling blocks in an IDS context, where, for example, the hospital is related to a for-profit management company. Violations of these guidelines may cause the bonds to become retroactively taxable unless certain actions are taken. Often the bonds must be repaid immediately. Sometimes, the repayment can be made only by paying the bondholders a substantial premium.

PROVIDER LICENSURE LAWS AND CORPORATE PRACTICE OF MEDICINE

Unlike antitrust, fraud and abuse, and tax considerations, licensure of health care providers is exclusively under the purview of each state. Generally, all providers of health care services must obtain a license, but certain exceptions may apply. For example, in some states certain free-standing facilities such as ambulatory surgery centers may not require licensure if they are wholly owned or controlled by physicians. Licensure is generally the cornerstone for reimbursement; Medicare and Medicaid require certification, which may be granted on the basis of licensure.

Some states prohibit the "corporate practice of medicine." These statutes generally preclude a business or nonlicensed corporation from providing medical services. These prohibitions may affect the employment of physicians and impact the methodology of reimbursement or remuneration for services rendered.

In the IDS context, state laws on the corporate practice of medicine can be very influential in structuring the means of physician practice acquisitions to employ all physicians in a professional corporation (PC). The hospital, or IDS, may not own stock in a PC, resulting in structures that have long-term management services agreements between the IDS and the PC or structures where a "friendly" physician owns the stock of the PC, but certain protections for oversight by the IDS are built into the structure.

Recent IRS rulings have allowed PCs closely affiliated with a tax-exempt IDS to obtain tax-exempt status. Exemption rested on the de facto control by the hospital component of the IDS and the fact that the PCs were direct providers of care with a strong charity care policy.

INSURANCE LICENSURE

State insurance regulators are currently pondering the question of whether risk-bearing providers, including IDSs, are in the business of insurance or merely parties to an insurance contract. The concern is that if provider entities are accepting global risk on a prepaid basis (capitation), they are in the business of insurance and must comply with insurance licensure laws.

In the insurance context, regulatory concerns relate primarily to consumer protection, including the solvency of the insurer, continuity of benefits, adequacy of handling consumer complaints, and so on. The National Association of Insurance Commissioners (NAIC) has taken the position that an IDS assuming "downstream risk" under contract with a licensed entity, such as an HMO, is not itself subject to direct regulation; the regulation of the licensed insurer is sufficient to ensure the level of public protection required by public policy. However, where there is no licensed entity involved and the IDS assumes risk directly from the ultimate purchaser of services (for example, a self-insured employer), the NAIC believes that regulatory oversight is required.

In spite of this pronouncement by the NAIC, most states have not explicitly adopted the proposed NAIC policy. Some states have specifically adopted their own regulatory requirements for risk-bearing IDSs even when the IDS is accepting downstream risk from licensed insurers. A health care executive should understand the regulatory environment with respect to the business of insurance in the state(s) in which the IDS operates and should be particularly cautious with respect to such requirements if the IDS is assuming risk in direct contracts with self-insured employers or other nonlicensed entities.

OTHER ISSUES

Other state and federal laws may impact the development or activities of an IDS. For example, employment and labor laws may be relevant, depending on the particular activities of the IDS. Pension plan concerns are often of great importance to physicians affiliating with an IDS. A physician practice is more likely to have a more generous retirement plan than a hospital because of the range of employees and compensation levels. As a result, there may be affiliated structures in the IDS; if so, they must meet certain requirements under the Employee Retirement Income Security Act for affiliated service groups or leased employees in order to ensure that the tax qualification of the plan will be maintained. Furthermore, other employment and labor laws, including the National Labor Relations Act, the Age Discrimination in Employment Act of 1967, and the Americans with Disabilities Act, may be relevant to a particular IDS undertaking.

Federal and state securities laws may also be applicable in an IDS development project if the IDS is going to sell economic interests. Membership interests in nonprofit corporations are usually not regarded as securities, but the facts and circumstances of transferability, distributions, and termination rights should be evaluated with that possibility in mind. Even if the interests do meet the definition of securities, exemptions are available from registration requirements under certain circumstances. A health care executive considering an activity that might involve the issuance of securities should review the structure to analyze whether exemptions are available.

Any particular IDS undertaking may involve other legal considerations such as intellectual property laws, real estate, environmental, or certificate-of-need laws. Such laws should be considered in the specific context of the IDS project.

CONCLUSION

Myriad legal issues must be considered in the development, maintenance, or expansion of an IDS. Health care executives should consult with legal counsel expert in the foregoing areas to ensure that the activities undertaken by the IDS are structured and managed with minimal legal risk.

Notes

1. Note that although vertical integration may pass antitrust muster, integration of providers for the purpose of generating referrals may pose fraud and abuse problems.

2. In general, acquisitions may be reportable under Hart-Scott-Rodino if (1) either party to the transaction is engaged in interstate commerce, (2) the acquiree has assets of more than $10 million (sales or assets if the acquiree is a manufacturer) and the acquiror has sales or assets of more than $100 million, or the acquiree has sales or assets of more than $100 million and the acquiror has sales or assets of more than $10 million, and (3) the transaction amounts to more than $15 million.

3. Before relying on the risk-sharing arrangement exception, executives should verify its statutory validity, as the Clinton Administration in 1996 expressed its desire that Congress repeal the newest safe harbor.

Glossary

AAPCC: *See* **Average Adjusted Per Capita Cost.**

Academic medical center: A medical center that is affiliated with or part of an accredited medical school with an accredited medical residency training program.

Acute care hospital: A short-term general hospital that provides inpatient episodic care to patients for a period of less than a month.

Administrative services only (ASO): Provision of claims processing and related administrative services to a health plan, typically a self-insured employer plan. Generally the ASO contractor does not assume risk for the insured group and is not liable for the costs of providing care to a plan member.

Adverse selection: (1) A phenomenon in which health plan members generally use more services and are more expensive to care for than expected. (2) A situation in which a health plan attracts sicker-than-average members and has a disproportionate enrollment of high-risk individuals.

Affiliated: Associated by common control or agreement but not necessarily ownership.

Agency for Health Care Policy and Research (AHCPR): A branch of the U.S. Public Health Service under the Department of Health and Human Services that is responsible for conducting and/or fostering health services research regarding medical effectiveness, patient outcomes, quality of care, and cost of care, and for creating state-of-the-art medical practice guidelines to identify how injuries and illnesses can be most effectively prevented, diagnosed, and clinically managed. AHCPR is also charged with using the resulting data to promote improvement in clinical practice and in the organization, financing, and delivery of care.

AHCPR: *See* **Agency for Health Care Policy and Research.**

Aligned incentives: Financial incentives that encourage stakeholders to achieve shared organizational goals. In an integrated health care system, incentives should be aligned for different provider organizations, different health care professionals, and between health care and financing components.

Alliance: (1) A voluntary organization of independent institutions, organizations, health systems, health plans, or business coalitions that share a common goal and join together without single ownership. (2) A public or private purchasing coalition formed to consolidate and organize the purchase of health insurance coverage for groups and/or individuals.

ALOS: *See* **Average Length of Stay.**

Alternate delivery system: A term formerly applied to HMOs and other managed care plans that once were regarded as an alternative to indemnity coverage. The prevalence of managed care plans has changed them from an alternative to a common type of delivery and financing of health care.

Alternative care: Medical treatment that is a medically justified substitute for inpatient hospitalization. An example is outpatient as opposed to inpatient surgery. As alternative care becomes part of standard medical practice, the term is used less frequently.

Ambulatory care: (1) Health services provided to patients who can move around on their own and are not bedridden. (2) Medical care provided outside an inpatient or residential care facility, such as outpatient care. The term applies to a broad range of services including diagnosis and treatment, rehabilitation care, routine preventive care, episodic acute care provided in physician offices and urgent care centers, and day surgery applied in free-standing facilities. In integrated health care systems that accept financial risk, providers are encouraged to recommend ambulatory care rather than inpatient care when medically appropriate.

Any willing provider (AWP) laws: Legislation requiring managed care plans to accept into their networks any provider willing to agree to the network's conditions. AWP laws are state specific.

ASO: *See* **Administrative services only.**

Average adjusted per capita cost (AAPCC): The basis of payment formula currently used for Medicare HMO risk plans.

Average length of stay (ALOS): The average number of days that patients are hospitalized. The term is sometimes used as a comparative measure of the severity of illness of a hospital's patient load or of a hospital's efficiency.

AWP: *See* **Any willing provider laws.**

Benefit package: Collection of specific services or benefits that a managed care plan is obligated to provide under the terms of its contracts with subscriber groups and individuals.

Business coalition: A local or regional group of employers, insurers, labor union representatives, and sometimes provider representatives who join to discuss and disseminate information on health care issues. Coalition members may also collect, analyze, and share health services and utilization information, conduct patient satisfaction and other surveys, compare health plans, and engage in group purchasing of health coverage for their employees.

Capitation: (1) A flat rate per person, paid in advance, for providing specified care to a health plan member for a specific length of time—for example, an amount paid per member per month to a primary care practitioner for the entire range of services that member may require for that month, regardless of how much service is actually required or rendered. Specialist physicians as well as primary care practitioners can be capitated. (2) A flat rate per student paid to medical schools by the federal government to help support medical education. *See also* **Per member per month.**

Carve-out: A strategy used by some managed care plans and/or purchasers of health insurance (for example, employers and other insured groups) to separately insure and/or manage specific services. Carve-outs are often high-cost or specialty services or services for which guidelines frequently change. Examples are mental health, substance abuse, dental, and pharmacy.

Case management: (1) Systematic organization and coordination of health services and resources done by providers and/or managed care plans and/or outside vendors to optimize clinical outcomes and manage risk. (2) Process by which patients in need of medical care are matched with providers and services to bring about the best result for the patient with the most efficient use of services, at an acceptable level of cost. The term has historically referred to complex and high-cost cases. With the growing prevalence of managed care, providers and health care systems that accept financial risk may use case management to promote health and wellness as well as to manage illness when it occurs.

Chemical dependency: Substance abuse or addiction such as drug abuse, alcoholism and alcohol abuse, and nicotine addiction.

Claim: (1) Request for payment under an insurance policy. (2) Submission of an itemized bill for services or covered items provided to an insured person. (3) The bill itself.

Clinical algorithm: A method of describing a clinical practice guideline that uses a structured flowchart of if-then decision steps and preferred clinical management pathways. *See also* **Clinical practice guidelines.**

Clinical integration: Methods by which integrated health care systems can mass customize the delivery of care so it is delivered and measured in ways that have common efficiencies but meet individual needs. The term encompasses existence of a continuum of care, coordination of care, disease management, communication, smooth transfer of information and medical records, elimination of duplicative processes and procedures, and efficient use of resources.

Clinical practice guidelines: Standards for clinical practice for particular treatments and procedures created by comparing the current practices of physicians. *See also* **Clinical algorithm.**

Closed formulary: A specified list of prescription drugs, generally compiled by a health plan's pharmacy and therapeutics committee, that are covered by the plan's benefit package. Exceptions from the list are generally not allowed without prior consultation between the prescribing physician and the medical director of the health plan. Health care providers as well as health plans can set policies regarding closed formularies. *See also* **Open formulary.**

Closed-panel HMO: HMO that provides care to enrollees by a restricted panel of physicians who are organized as a staff- or group-model HMO. *See also* **Group-model HMO; Staff-model HMO.**

CMP: *See* **Competitive medical plan.**

Coinsurance: The percentage of an insurance claim that an insured person must pay before reimbursement applies. For example, in an 80/20 plan, the plan member pays 20 percent of the claim and the plan pays 80 percent.

Community hospital: A privately owned acute care general hospital.

Community rating: (1) Method of setting premium rates that takes into account only the aggregate projected experience of an entire health plan population, not the projected experience of an individual or employer group. (2) Method of premium setting in which an individual or group's premium rate is based on the actual or anticipated cost of care for all members of a health plan in a specific service area. (3) Method of premium setting that reflects the experience of an entire population or community (for example, city, metropolitan area, state, region, nation). *See also* **Experience rating.**

Competitive medical plan (CMP): HMO-like provider group that meets specific criteria allowing it to participate in Medicare risk contracting but that is not federally qualified as an HMO. Examples are HMOs that are state-qualified, and capitated multi-specialty medical groups.

Concurrent review: A determination made by a health plan at the time care is being sought that the care is medically necessary and should be continued. It often applies to continued hospital stay. Concurrent review is an adjunct to precertification and is usually but not always performed over the telephone.

Continuous quality improvement (CQI): A management and quality control approach that emphasizes a continuous process of meeting and, over time, exceeding specified performance goals related to consumer needs and expectations. The goal of CQI is to examine systems for systemic flaws, not just individual errors, and improve average performance by measuring, analyzing, and reducing or eliminating variation in processes and products. *See also* **Total quality management.**

Continuum of care: The full scope of services needed to encourage good health and treat illness when it occurs. Components include health education and wellness, primary care, acute care management, tertiary and quaternary care, supportive care (home care), subacute care, long-term care, rehabilitation, and skilled nursing care.

Co-payment: A specified out-of-pocket amount that a health plan member must pay for a specific service provided under the plan. Common examples are a fixed dollar amount per physician office visit or per drug prescription.

Cost-based reimbursement: A method by which third parties reimburse providers for the provision of care. The amount of payment is based on the cost to the provider. Historically, cost-based reimbursement has contributed to the rise and growth rate of health care costs.

Cost contract: Under the rules of the Tax Equity and Fiscal Responsibility Act (TEFRA) rules, an HMO or CMP can contract with Medicare to provide care to members under the limits of Medicare-specified cost limits. This arrangement is often selected by participating plans in areas where provider costs are lower than average in comparison with other regions. *See also* **Risk contract.**

Cost effectiveness: The degree to which a service meets a specified goal at an acceptable cost, where the emphasis is first on meeting the goal and only secondarily on cost. It is not the same as getting the best results for the price, an approach that emphasizes cost and makes results secondary.

Cost sharing: A situation in which the employer and health plan member or insured person share the cost of coverage. The sharing may apply to a premium and/or to deductibles, coinsurance, co-payments, and amounts exceeding a plan's payment limits.

Coverage: Provision of insurance under a policy to cover specific reimbursable costs; in health insurance, coverage means financing of health services obtained by insured persons. Coverage can enable but not guarantee provision of health services; provision is also dependent on availability and access of services.

Coverage option: A rider that specifies coverage beyond that required by an insurance policy. The additional coverage is not automatic and may be added at the discretion of the insured group or individual at an additional cost.

CPT: *See* **Current procedural terminology.**

CQI: *See* **Continuous quality improvement.**

Credentialing: The formal process of examining professional credentials, abilities, and qualifications of physicians and other practitioners before approving them for participation in a hospital staff or the provider panel of a health plan or other organized delivery system. The professionals under review must be licensed and meet other specified criteria such as certification in a particular specialty or evidence of continuing professional education. Economic factors such as a clinician's historic practice patterns in providing care to a specific group of patients can be part of the credentialing process.

Current Procedural Terminology (CPT): A classification system of terminology and coding developed by the American Medical Association. It is used to describe, code, and report medical services and procedures. The fourth edition is known as *CPT-4*.

Days per thousand: (1) A health plan's total number of inpatient days per thousand plan members for a specific 12-month period. (2) A hospital's average number of inpatient days per thousand inpatients.

Deductible: The out-of-pocket cost that a health plan member must pay per year before the health insurance coverage applies. The deductible is usually expressed as a set dollar amount per benefit year.

Diagnosis-related groups (DRGs): (1) The classification system developed for Medicare that categorizes a hospitalization according to the patient's primary diagnosis and assigns a DRG code. (2) A per case reimbursement mechanism for hospital stays, developed for Medicare but used by other payers, that pays a flat rate per diagnosis according to the DRG category to which the patient's case is assigned. The payment is usually paid per episode or hospital stay regardless of how many days the patient actually stays in the hospital.

Direct contracting: An agreement between a purchaser (for example, employer, union health and welfare fund) and providers to render care to employees and/or retirees without the involvement of an insurer or health plan. Under such arrangements, a third-party administrator often handles administrative functions such as enrollment and claims payment.

Disability management: A strategy directed toward preventing the occurrence of a disabling illness or injury, ensuring safe and appropriate return to work after the occurrence and treatment, and promoting optimal possible functioning for the ill or injured person.

Discharge planning: Act or process of evaluating the need for and arranging necessary post-hospital care and services in advance of the patient's discharge or release. The planning can be done in any inpatient facility (for example, acute and tertiary hospitals, nursing homes, skilled nursing facility). As the function of case management becomes more prevalent, it often but not always includes discharge planning.

Discounted fee-for-service: A discount from the usual fee-for-service payment or fee schedule payment paid to a provider. This method of payment is often but not always used in exchange for a promise of volume.

Disease management: The process of treating a specific illness, injury, or condition by studying the disease life cycle and then designing appropriate interventions for each stage of the condition. The program manages each patient's care against the normative model of care developed by the process. It also targets potentially affected patients and takes a comprehensive approach to treating them, including but not limited to patient education and training in self-care, so that the disease is optimally managed over time.

DRG: *See* **Diagnosis-related groups.**

Dual choice: A health benefit offered by an employment group that permits eligibles of the group to voluntarily choose from different health plan options. The choice often includes an indemnity-type plan offered by the employer's primary insurer and a managed care plan.

Eligibility verification: The process of confirming a person's eligibility for coverage under a health plan, usually before health care services are provided or a prescription is filled.

Employee Retirement Income Security Act of 1974 (ERISA): The federal pension reform law that also regulates other employee benefits and exempts self-funded (self-insured) employer plans from state regulation, with the exception of workers' compensation plans. Because over half of U.S. companies are self-insured, ERISA can be a major obstacle to state-based health care reform initiatives. *See also* **Self-insured plan.**

Employer group: (1) All plan members or enrollees covered through a given employer. (2) Component of the private or commercial enrollment of a health plan, as opposed to enrollees sponsored by public payers; commercial enrollment in a health plan that is not self-insured usually includes many different employer groups.

Enrollment: (1) The act or process of joining a health plan. (2) Membership of insured persons in an HMO or point-of-service plan.

EPO: *See* **Exclusive provider organization.**

Exclusive provider organization (EPO): Type of health plan that requires members to use providers in its provider network to qualify for benefit coverage. EPOs usually do not capitate providers and generally do not have an HMO license.

Experience rating: A method of determining insurance rates that takes into account the previous experience and claims history of the person or entity to be insured. *See also* **Community rating.**

Fee-for-service (FFS): Method of payment in which each service provided to patients is associated with a corresponding fee that is paid to the provider.

Fee schedule: Defines a fixed reimbursement level for particular services rather than basing payment on physician charge profiles. The fees can be based on relative value units, such as the resource-based relative value (RBRVS) scale adopted by Medicare. Other examples of fee schedules are the California RBRVS and the McGraw-Hill RBRVS.

FFS: *See* **Fee-for-service.**

For-profit: Operated for the benefit of shareholders, who receive a share of the profits earned. For-profit organizations can be privately owned or publicly traded organizations. They pay both federal and state taxes.

Full-risk contract: *See* **Global capitation.**

Functional integration: The extent to which key support functions and activities are coordinated across operating units to add the greatest overall value to the system. Examples are human resources, support services, culture, strategic planning, quality assurance, marketing, information systems, and financial management.

Gatekeeper: A health care professional who coordinates, manages, and authorizes all health care services provided to a covered beneficiary. The professional may be a physician, nurse, social worker, or physician's assistant. Managed care plans often designate and capitate gatekeepers in order to control costs.

Global capitation: Also known as full capitation, this is a single payment made by a health plan to an institutional provider or provider organization that is responsible for the full scope of services to be provided to plan members. The recipient of the capitation payment is responsible for dividing the payment among individual practitioners and institutional or organizational providers. The provider must also pay other providers who provide services that it cannot provide.

Global payment: Prospectively defined limits on spending for some portion of the health care industry, such as hospital operating budgets or both hospital and physician services.

Group coverage: Insurance coverage obtained through an employer-sponsored plan, wherein the insured person is part of the employer group.

Group-model HMO: HMO that contracts with one or more independent group practices that provide health services exclusively to HMO patients. *See also* **Closed-panel HMO; staff-model HMO.**

Group practice: (1) A contractual arrangement in which two or more physicians practice medicine together in a collegial fashion, share the assets of the practice, and care for and share liability for each other's patients. (2) The basis of group-model and network-model HMOs.

HCFA: *See* **Health Care Financing Administration.**

Health care delivery system: (1) An organized system that provides health care services in a given service area or region. (2) The entire health care infrastructure that provides health services to people of a given nation; may be referred to as *the* health care delivery system (national) rather than *a* delivery system (local).

Health Care Financing Administration (HCFA): The federal agency responsible for administering Medicare and overseeing the states' administration of Medicaid.

Health maintenance organization (HMO): (1) State-licensed health plan that offers prepaid, comprehensive coverage for hospital and physician services, manages care, and restricts members to use of only providers affiliated with the plan. Members enroll for a specified period. Other HMO features are provider risk-sharing and prepayment of per member per month premiums. (2) Type of prepaid, state-licensed health plan that combines the financing or insurance aspect of coverage with the actual provision of medical care.

Health Plan Employer Data and Information Set (HEDIS): A data set of health plan performance indicators and other information created and updated by the National Committee for Quality Assurance. At the outset, there were different versions for commercial, Medicare, and Medicaid plans; these will be blended together. HEDIS provides health plans with a uniform format for reporting data to purchasers and the public so that comparisons can be made. Point-of-service plans report HEDIS data if they are HMO-based; PPOs and indemnity plans do not report. *See also* **National Committee for Quality Assurance.**

Health plan member: (1) Known as an enrollee, a person who is covered under a health plan. (2) The person in whose name the insurance policy is issued, as opposed to that person's covered dependents and spouse.

Health promotion: Activities sponsored by a health plan, provider, and/or employer that are aimed at encouraging and helping people improve their health and well-being. Examples are patient education programs, wellness activities, health fairs, and medical literature search services.

Health risk assessment: Analysis of the health status and risk factors affecting a particular patient or health plan member.

HEDIS: *See* **Health Plan Employer Data and Information Set.**

HMO: *See* **Health maintenance organization.**

Home health agency: Visiting nurse association or other home care vendor certified to deal with the Medicare program and beneficiaries who require home care services.

Home health care: Home health services provided in a patient's home as an alternative to inpatient or nursing home care, provided by an agency licensed by the state to render such care. Home care is provided to patients who are under a physician's care, homebound for medical reasons, and therefore physically unable to obtain the necessary services on an ambulatory basis. Services may include nursing care; social and support services; physical, speech, occupational, or inhalation therapy; home infusion therapy, including chemotherapy; or the provision of durable medical equipment required for eligible homebound patients.

Horizontal integration: The consolidation of like organizations or business ventures under a single corporate management to produce synergy, reduce redundancies and duplication of efforts or products, and achieve economies of scale while increasing market share. Examples in health care include alliances, IPAs, and mergers among hospitals or health plans.

Hospice: A multidisciplinary program that provides medical care (including nursing care and pain and symptom management), counseling, and support services for terminally ill patients, and counseling and bereavement services for their families. The program must be licensed or certified to operate within its jurisdiction and must be directed and coordinated by medical professionals. Hospice care may be provided on an ambulatory and home care basis or in a residential care or inpatient facility. Eligible patients typically must be certified by their physicians as having a terminal diagnosis and six months or less to live, although the time element varies. Acquired immune deficiency syndrome (AIDS) programs often have a hospice component without a time factor.

Incentive compensation: Compensation that includes financial rewards and/or penalties for specified performance. Compensation may be modified by incentives or totally dependent on them. For example, under capitation, the method of payment encourages providers to practice medicine in ways that facilitate achievement of utilization and cost targets. But the incentive is indirect because the amount of the capitation payment does not increase with the amount or type of service rendered. In contrast, when money is withheld from compensation with potential repayment based on specified criteria, the incentive is directly related to desired performance.

Indemnity plan: (1) A traditional insurance plan that reimburses the insured person when a claim is made. (2) In health care, a fee-for-service plan that pays for services rendered.

Independent practice association (IPA): (1) An association of independent physicians who have joined together to negotiate managed care contracts. (2) A provider network consisting entirely of independent physicians who practice in their own offices rather than at a clinic site.

Integrated health care system: Organized delivery (and sometimes financing) that provides comprehensive health services to a defined population. In an integrated system, the different parts of the system work together to achieve economies of scale and other synergies to a degree not achieved by other delivery mechanisms. The term is often misused to describe any system that combines some aspects of delivery and financing.

Intermediate care facility: A facility or distinct part of an inpatient facility that is licensed to provide care to patients who do not require the level and intensity of care provided by a hospital or skilled nursing facility but who, because of their physical or mental conditions, require care and services beyond custodial care (room and board).

IPA: *See* **Independent practice association.**

Long-term care: The range of health services provided to chronically ill, disabled, or retarded persons in an inpatient setting or a residential, home care, or ambulatory care basis, or any combination thereof. The care extends from over a month to years. The inpatient facilities may include specialty hospitals, rehabilitation care facilities, and nursing homes.

Malcolm Baldrige National Quality Award: Administered by the U.S. Department of Commerce and named for a past Secretary of Commerce, this prestigious award goes annually to companies that meet the rigorous standards of the program for the manufacture and sale of products and services. Integrated health care systems and other health care organizations can use the standards to define their quality goals. They are also eligible to receive the award.

Managed care: (1) A systematic approach to providing organized health care services that manages the cost and use of services while measuring and monitoring the performance of the plan and its providers. The goal is to provide cost-effective care to plan members. (2) Health plans such as HMOs, PPOs, point-of-service plans, and occasionally managed indemnity plans.

Management service organization (MSO): An organization formed by one or more physician group practices to manage their medical practices. Typical responsibilities of an MSO are site selection and maintenance, furnishing, equipment purchase and maintenance, administrative services, and information systems.

Market area: A targeted geographic area in which the principal market potential is located. It may or may not be the same as an HMO's formally defined service area.

Market penetration: In health insurance, the percentage of all insured individuals in a given geographic market or service area who are enrolled in a specific health plan or type of health plan (for example, HMO, PPO, point-of-service plan). The general term *HMO penetration* refers to the percentage of the insured persons in a market who are enrolled in any HMO operating in that market.

Medicaid managed care: A range of programs that apply managed care principles to Medicaid programs. They may include HMO risk contracts, primary care case management, or cost contracts. Medicaid is administered and partially funded by each state, and many states have received federal waivers to develop their programs

Medical necessity: Care clinically judged to be required to preserve the life or health of the patient, with the expectation that the benefits of such care generally outweigh the risks to the patient. In a managed care environment, health plans and providers determine medical necessity.

Medicare risk contract: *See* **Risk contract.**

Member month: Unit of volume measurement indicating the length of time that the member is enrolled in an HMO, regardless of whether or not the member seeks and receives health care during that time. Many internal operating statistics for HMOs are expressed in terms of member months. *See also* **Capitation; Per member per month.**

Mixed-model HMO: HMO that uses any combination of staff physicians, group practices, IPAs, and/or solo practitioners for its provider network.

MSO: *See* **Management service organization.**

Multihospital system: Two or more hospitals owned, operated under lease or contract, or sponsored by a central organization that provides overall direction.

Multi-option plan: A health plan that offers employees the option of enrolling under one of several types of coverage, usually an HMO, a PPO, or an indemnity plan.

National Committee for Quality Assurance (NCQA): A not-for-profit organization founded in 1990 to define quality, develop ways to measure it, and share information with purchasers and the public. Its health plan accreditation is available to the public. Working first with private employers and later with the public sector, NCQA has developed HEDIS criteria that purchasers and ultimately customers can use to select health plans. *See also* **Health Plan Employer Data and Information Set.**

NCQA: *See* **National Committee for Quality Assurance.**

Network-model HMO: HMO that contracts with two or more independent group practices that provide health services to HMO patients and patients covered by other payers.

Not-for-profit: Operated for the benefit of the community, rather than shareholders, under the ownership of a private corporation. Profits are retained within the institution or organization for future use and growth or for new programs. The organization or institution must meet requirements specified by federal and state tax laws and regulations to gain legal designation and accompanying exemption from federal and state taxes. Typically the institution or organization has public representation on its board of trustees and depends on philanthropy for initial or some continuing funding.

Open-ended HMO: HMO that permits its enrollees to receive some health services from physicians and/or hospitals that are outside the HMO's provider network, in exchange for higher out-of-pocket costs for the plan member. In an open-ended HMO, the member is automatically enrolled in the HMO and has little or no out-of-pocket costs for care received from in-network providers. *See also* **Point-of-service plan.**

Open enrollment: A period during which people in an employer group may join or change health plans without penalty. Open enrollment occurs a few weeks or months prior to the start of a new benefit year.

Open formulary: A list of preferred prescription drugs that a health plan's participating providers are encouraged to use in treatment. Exceptions are allowed and covered under the plan but may require a higher co-payment, depending on the plan member's specific benefit package. *See also* **Closed formulary.**

Open-panel HMO: (1) An HMO in which participating physicians provide care in their own offices as independent practitioners. They are not salaried employees of the health plan. An IPA-type HMO is one example. (2) An HMO in which enrollees can self-refer to specialists without authorization by primary care practitioners.

Organized delivery system: A generic name for networks of health care delivery organizations and/or institutions that provide or arrange for a broad range of coordinated care for a defined population; are clinically and financially accountable for the outcomes and health status of the population(s) served; and own, are owned by, or are closely allied with a health plan. The organized systems and their affiliated practitioners should be placed at financial risk by the health plans with which they have relationships (ownership or contractual). Nonetheless, many organized delivery systems are not yet at financial risk, although they do have a continuum of care, accountability, and connection(s) to a health plan(s).

Outcome study: A systematic study undertaken across a group of patients to observe the effects of treatment for a specific illness, injury, or condition. The study may or may not take into account the comparative cost/benefit of competing treatments.

Outcomes research: The study of the health effects that patients experience as a result of medical care. The results may include short- and/or long-term effects on patients.

Out-of-area benefits: The benefits that a health plan provides to subscribers who are outside the plan's geographic limits when they become ill. Emergency care is usually included. When enrollees use out-of-area benefits, they are expected to notify the plan and to seek in-area care for follow-up medical management.

Out-of-pocket cost: The portion of medical costs that a plan member or insured person must pay for receiving care as opposed to the portion paid by the plan. Out-of-pocket costs may include co-payments, deductibles, and coinsurance amounts as well as balance billing, premium contributions, and uncovered services.

Package pricing: A payment method that combines the fees for professional and institutional services associated with a procedure into a single amount. Also known as service bundling or global pricing, package pricing sets the price of the bundled procedures and therefore implicitly controls the volume of services provided as part of the global service.

Participating provider: A provider who has contracted with a health plan to provide medical services to covered persons. The provider may be a hospital, pharmacy, other facility, physician, or other clinician (for example, physical therapist) who has contractually accepted the terms and conditions as set forth by the health plan.

PCP: *See* **Primary care practitioner.**

Peer review: Evaluation of a physician's performance by other physicians, usually within the same geographic area and medical specialty.

Penetration: The percentage of business that an HMO or other health plan is able to capture in a particular subscriber group or in the market area as a whole. For example, enrolling 10 members out of 100 eligibles yields a 10 percent penetration.

Per diem: A set per-day rate paid by a health plan for hospitalizations or other inpatient or residential care. The amount can be service-specific (for example, medical/surgical, pediatric, obstetrical, mental health/substance abuse) or an average amount for all services.

Per member per month (PMPM): A unit of premium payment for a managed care plan, literally a flat rate per member. *See also* **Capitation; Member month.**

PHO: *See* **Physician-hospital organization.**

Physician-hospital organization (PHO): A legal entity that includes at least one hospital and at least one physician organization, such as a group practice or an IPA, and is empowered to negotiate or contract with health plans on behalf of both the hospital(s) and the physicians. The PHO may or may not be legally structured as a joint venture between physicians and a hospital or multihospital system.

PMPM: *See* **Per member per month.**

Point-of-service (POS) plan: A type of fee-for-service plan that allows members to choose at the time they need care whether to receive it from a provider within the plan's network or from a provider outside the network. If the member opts to seek care from an out-of-network provider, the out-of-pocket cost to the member is greater. Open-ended HMOs may have POS-like features. *See also* **Open-ended HMO.**

Population-based care: (1) Provision of health services that focuses on the current and long-term needs of populations within a health plan or geographic area rather than only on individual patients' requirements. (2) Care that uses population-based measures of health status to ascertain progress and providers' or health plans' performance. Population-based care may focus on the entire enrolled population or classify subsets of the population according to target group characteristics such as demographics, geographic area, clinical conditions, and risk factors/characteristics.

POS: *See* **Point-of-service plan.**

PPO: *See* **Preferred provider organization.**

Precertification: The process by which a health plan approves coverage and the use of services prior to the fact (for example, approval for hospitalization in advance of the admission). Established clinical protocols often assist the reviewer in determining authorization of an admission and length of stay. *See also* **Prior authorization.**

Preferred provider organization (PPO): A type of fee-for-service health plan in which members may obtain care either from an affiliated network of physicians, hospitals, and other providers or from any other providers they choose. However, if a member sees an affiliated provider within the network, the member's co-payments and deductible costs are lower than if the member goes outside the network for care. In general, PPOs pay discounted provider fees. They may have incentives for providers and plan members and some degree of utilization management.

Premium: (1) The cost of obtaining health insurance coverage. (2) The payment for an insurance policy, which may be paid on a monthly, quarterly, or annual basis. (3) The premium rate.

Prepaid group practice: (1) A physician group practice that provides services to members who pay a flat rate in advance, per person, for a given time period. (2) The antecedent of group-model HMOs. (3) Another name for a group-model HMO.

Primary care: Basic or general health care typically provided by physicians and nurse practitioners who specialize in family or general practice, pediatrics, and/or internal medicine. Sometimes obstetrics/gynecologist specialists are included.

Primary care case management: Managed care arrangements in which primary care providers receive a per capita management fee to coordinate a patient's care in addition to the reimbursement for medical services provided. Sometimes providers are at financial risk. In many states, Medicaid managed care programs use this approach to managing patient care.

Primary care practitioner (PCP): A physician or nurse specialist who provides most of patients' routine medical care and who is trained in general or family practice, internal medicine, pediatrics, or obstetrics and gynecology.

Prior authorization: The process of obtaining approval for coverage and use of a medical service. Without such prior authorization, the service is not covered. *See also* **Precertification.**

Profiling: Statistical techniques used to describe the practice of physicians and other health care professionals. The purpose is to identify those who overutilize or underutilize services as compared with benchmarks. The purpose of profiling is to improve the quality of care through education and feedback.

Proprietary: *See* **For-profit.**

Protocol: The plan or outline of a scientific experiment, study, or medical treatment. *See also* clinical practice guidelines and clinical algorithm.

Provider: An individual health care practitioner, medical group, or institution/organization that renders health care services.

Provider-sponsored organization: Willingness of health care providers, usually physicians and/or hospitals, to assume financial risk so they can contract directly with purchasers without going through insurers as a middle party. Recent federal legislation allows such arrangements under certain conditions. Many health plans and insurance companies oppose the concept because they believe it will have a negative impact on their roles in the health care system.

PSO: *See* **Provider-sponsored organization.**

QA: *See* **Quality assurance program.**

Quality assurance (QA) program: In health care, a set of activities intended to determine and monitor the quality of care provided to patients. Because it focuses on identifying and preventing inappropriate care or fraud and abuse, quality assurance is generally considered a more passive and rudimentary activity than quality management or quality improvement programs, which involve active intervention in routine care and in exceptions to the norm.

Rate setting: The setting of hospital service rates or health plan premium rates by a governmental agency or commission, usually a state agency. Rate setting may or may not include the setting of local Medicare and/or Medicaid rates, depending on whether or not the state has an all-payer program waiver from one or both of these programs.

RBRVS: *See* **Resource-based relative value scale.**

Rehabilitation hospital: A specialized facility dedicated to the treatment of patients requiring longer-term physical rehabilitation, along with counseling and support services, for which a prolonged stay in an acute-care hospital or nursing home is inappropriate; the goal of rehabilitation care is to help the patient recover as much mobility, function, and independence as possible given the illness or injury. Rehabilitation care often follows severe or traumatic injury.

Reinsurance: Excess insurance coverage through which the at-risk entity (for example, health plan, capitated provider or organization, employer) passes on some or all of its risk to the reinsurer. The purpose is to protect the insured from insolvency due to unexpected catastrophic cases. *See also* **Stop-loss coverage.**

Residential care facility: (1) A facility that provides food, shelter, laundry, and other services, possibly but not necessarily including medical care, to unrelated residents. Examples are homes for the aged and boarding homes for sheltered care. (2) Regarding mental health or behavioral care, a treatment facility where patients, usually ambulatory, live and receive care in a nonhospital setting.

Resource-based relative value scale (RBRVS): A scale that measures the relative work effort and resources used by physicians for different procedures and different levels of office visits. The scale was created for the Medicare program by William Hsiao and colleagues at the Harvard School of Public Health.

Retrospective review: A determination made by a health plan, after the fact, of the need for medical treatment for a specific episode of care. As state insurance commissioners become more concerned with protecting consumers from potential abuses by managed care plans, some of them are questioning the appropriateness of health plan review procedures.

Risk: (1) In insurance, the amount of uncertainty involved in predicting loss expense or claims under a specific policy. (2) The degree to which an insured person or entity is likely to make a claim; the more likely the claim and the higher the associated expense, the higher the risk to the insurer issuing the policy. Low-risk insureds are those for whom the anticipated risk can be reliably predicted and whose anticipated claims are infrequent and of low cost. High-risk insureds are those for whom claims are expected to be high in total cost or for whom risk cannot be reliably calculated.

Risk contract: (1) Also known as a TEFRA risk contract, an agreement between an HMO or CMP and Medicare (as authorized by the federal Tax Equity and Fiscal Responsibility Act) to provide all specified care and coverage to Medicare members at a prepaid flat rate per member per month; the plan assumes the risk that the flat rate may not cover all services required by a patient for a given month. (2) Any contract between a health plan and a provider wherein the provider accepts a flat rate for all care to be provided during a given period or for a given episode of care, thereby taking on risk. *See also* **Cost contract.**

Risk pool: Combining specific insured populations into a single large group to distribute risk over a larger number of insureds, avoid adverse selection, and lower the premium cost to higher-risk insureds.

Risk spreading: The act of distributing risk across a large group of insureds or health plans; the essence of pooling and of insurance itself.

Selective contracting: The practice of doing business with a limited number of contractors, usually according to predetermined criteria, to concentrate or increase market share for those contractors and increase the influence of the organization offering the contract.

Self-administered plan: One in which the employer or welfare fund handles claims administration and reimbursement without assistance from an insurer or other intermediary. Under such plans, some benefits may be insured or subcontracted and others may be self-funded. Often a third-party administrator is hired to handle administrative aspects of the plan.

Self-funding: *See* **Self-insured plan.**

Self-insured plan: An employee benefit, welfare, pension, or other insurance plan for which the employer has set aside funds and taken on the risk rather than passing on that risk to an insurer; all such plans that benefit employees and/or retirees are commonly known as ERISA plans because they are exempt from state regulation, except for workers' compensation laws. *See also* **Employee Retirement Income Security Act of 1974.**

Skilled nursing facility (SNF): A facility or distinct part of an institution that is separately licensed to provide 24-hour inpatient nursing care to patients who are under the supervision of a physician and require skilled nursing care for a prolonged convalescence or for a chronic illness or condition over a long period. An SNF must have an attending medical staff of one or more physicians.

SNF: *See* **Skilled nursing facility.**

Solo practitioner: An independent physician who practices alone rather than in a group practice.

Specialty care: (1) Health care services beyond primary care that are provided by physicians, nurse specialists, and other selected health practitioners. (2) Services beyond primary care for which health plan members must obtain a referral from their primary care practitioners and/or from the managed care plan to which they belong.

Specialty care practitioner: A physician or nurse trained in a specialty other than primary care; may also include allied health professionals as well as selected other nonphysician health care practitioners.

Staff-model HMO: HMO that delivers health services through a salaried physician group employed by the HMO. *See also* **Closed-panel HMO; Group-model HMO.**

Stop-loss coverage: A form of reinsurance purchased by a health plan or health care provider that is automatically triggered when a claim exceeds a specified dollar amount or ceiling per individual subscriber. Stop-loss coverage is one form of solvency protection often required for health plans by insurance regulators. *See also* **Reinsurance.**

Subscriber: An enrolled employee or nongroup individual/family covered by a health plan.

Surplus: (1) The funds remaining after all costs have been covered; the excess of revenues over expenditures in a budget. (2) In not-for-profit organizations, the equivalent of profit; this money would be used within the organization rather than distributed to shareholders.

Teaching hospital: A hospital that has an accredited medical residency training program and that may be affiliated with a medical school.

Third-party administrator (TPA): A company that processes claims and performs other administrative services for a health plan, usually a self-insured employer plan.

Total quality management (TQM): A methodology that uses concepts originally developed by W. Edwards Deming to study systems and processes to identify and improve sources of error, waste, or redundancy. *See also* **Continuous quality improvement.**

TPA: *See* **Third-party administrator.**

TQM: *See* **Total quality management.**

Triple-option plan: A range of health plan coverage options including indemnity coverage, a PPO or point-of-service plan, and an HMO, all offered to an insured group by the same insurer as a unified product. A triple-option plan should not be confused with an employee benefit program that merely offers three separate health plan choices.

Urgent care: Medical care for an injury or illness that requires prompt attention but is not life threatening. In recognition of the need to make urgent care available and accessible, many providers have set up freestanding facilities/programs expressly for this purpose.

Utilization: The use of medical care services.

Utilization management: (1) The active management of all aspects of the use of medical care, including but not limited to utilization review, to produce optimal clinical results for patients with best use of resources. (2) A comprehensive set of strategies and techniques aimed at ensuring appropriate allocation of health care resources, that is, use of health services that takes into account medical necessity, timeliness, efficiency, and cost.

Utilization rate: The rate at which medical care services are used. It is often expressed as a single number (for example, total annual admissions), a ratio (for example, hospital days per thousand), or as a percentage (for example, 25 percent cesarean-section rate).

Utilization review: A concurrent or retrospective process of determining whether or not the provision of care is medically necessary and effective and represents the best use of resources for a specific illness, injury, or condition. The purpose is to reduce or eliminate unnecessary, ineffective, and equivocal care (care for which the amount of benefit to the patient is not clear).

Vertical integration: (1) Linking the related production functions of individual organizations into a new organization under single ownership or management to provide a full range of related products and/or services. (2) In health care, the combination through ownership or contractual relationships of dissimilar institutional and/or organizational providers to provide a continuum of care. The health care delivery system can be linked with suppliers and producers. If vertical integration is advanced, health care delivery and financing may be combined.

Virtual integration: In health care, a method of simulating integrated delivery or vertical integration through the use of contracts and/or formal affiliations rather than ownership.

Visual integration: That which payers and consumers see and experience with respect to integrated health care systems. Examples include access to care regardless of location, centralized appointment scheduling, and coordinated clinical care.

Withhold: The amount of a primary care physician's capitation or fee-for-service payment that is withheld by the health plan until year-end and used either to pay for incentive payments/ bonuses to primary care practitioners or retained by the plan or medical group as a result of a greater than expected use of services.

Workers' compensation: A no-fault insurance system regulated by each state in which all employers must participate and under which workers are compensated by their employers for the costs of work-related injuries and illnesses. It consists of two components: medical and related costs, and lost wages and disability payments.

Index